Introduction

A ketogenic diet will slowly help you get rid of bad food habits. The processed food diet most people follow cause untimely cravings. There are people who feel quite restless if they don't have certain snacks or sweets every single day. This unhealthy food addiction can be very damning for the body and mostly consists of empty calories. The keto diet works for both lazy and disciplined people. It is up to you to decide if you want a strict or more easygoing keto diet. Some people like to work on instinct when considering the food they eat while others prefer specific markers set for what their meals should consist of. This adjustable aspect of the keto diet makes it suitable for all types of people. Once you start reducing the carbohydrates in your diet and eating more fats, you will slowly get your body accustomed to breaking off the carb addiction. This will help you lose fat and maintain a healthy weight long-term.

It is easy to stick to a keto diet because the main parts of the meal such as meat, fish, and vegetables are not prohibited. The diet is only difficult for those who are too dependent on bread or such starchy foods in their meals. People who are overweight usually have a problem staying motivated to continue a diet. This is why strict diets often result in failure, but the keto diet can be a bit simpler for you compared to these diets. Keep track of your results in the first couple of weeks where you will first lose water weight. Slowly you will see the fat shedding from all parts of your body. Progress will be the best motivation for you to stay on the diet long-term.

Keto Diet Bible (For Beginners):

A Guide To Keto Weight Loss, Recipes, Intermittent Fasting & Motivation For Men & Women.

Table Of Contents

Chapter 1: Ketogenic Diet Overview

The Basics of the Ketogenic Diet

Before reading this beginner's guide, you may not have heard much about the ketogenic diet so we are going to go over the absolute basics. Before we get started, it's important that you realize what the ketogenic diet is. If you are rolling your eyes at the thought of another diet, understand that this isn't just any diet. While it may be slightly difficult to start, you will be absolutely amazed at the changes it can bring to your life. At the end of the day, you are in charge of your health and the ketogenic diet can change your life the same way that it has for countless others.

Put simply, the ketogenic diet is based around foods that are high in fat and low in carbohydrates, similar to the Atkins diet. For the most part, this diet is used to help boost an individual's metabolism and, in turn, helping people lose weight! You may be thinking, "I've been taught my whole life that fat is bad for you", but the truth is that it's all about the type of fat you eat while on the diet.

You may also notice that your protein intake is higher than normal whilst on the ketogenic diet. This is not a bad thing because when you are consuming mostly fats and protein, your body will begin to use these sources as energy as opposed to when one's diet is filled with carbohydrates. When you change your diet in this way, your body enters what is known as the state of ketosis.

Before the ketogenic diet was used for weight loss, it was first developed in the 1920's and 1930's as a treatment for epilepsy. Instead of mainstream fasting, scientists wanted to develop an alternative to show success in epilepsy therapy. It's still used to help with epilepsy today, but as scientists have learned, there are many other incredible benefits which can help a number of different people. Eventually, the ketogenic diet was abandoned due to other more effective therapies developed to treat epilepsy, including new emerging medications.

The first study which claimed that fasting was a cure was done in 1911 in France. In this study, patients were asked to follow a fasting schedule in addition to a low-calorie, vegetarian diet. When people followed this diet, studies showed an increase in mental capabilities. These studies were continued into the 20th Century where scientists found that during a low carbohydrate, high fat, and moderate protein diet, the body entered a state of what we now know as ketosis.

However, it wasn't until the 1960's that research began to show that ketones could be produced by what are known as medium-chain triglycerides or MCTs. These MCTs can be transported to the liver quickly in an oil form. This means that people on the ketogenic diet are able to consume more proteins and carbohydrates compared to the original ketogenic diet while consuming MCT oil.

What is Ketosis?

As previously mentioned, the point of the ketogenic diet is to put your body into a state of ketosis so that you can begin to generate energy in a different manner, i.e., mostly by fat. Keep in mind, however, that this can only occur when a diet consists of few carbohydrates and while fasting. The good news is that many people are able to lose weight this way. On the other hand, some people find it difficult to enter this state and maintain a lifestyle with ketosis.

The word "keto" comes from the word "ketones" which are small molecules that the body is able to use as fuel. These are produced when your blood sugar becomes lower in supply. You are able to lower your blood sugar by eating fewer carbohydrates, higher fat concentrations, and a moderate amount of protein. These ketones (fuel) are produced in the liver from the fats you will be eating on this diet. However, the brain is not able to function off fat alone. This is why your body converts these fats into ketones.

Today, there is a belief that your brain needs carbohydrates to function properly, however, scientific studies have shown that this isn't necessarily true. In fact, studies have shown that your brain can work just as well on ketones as it does with your current diet, if not better while on the ketogenic diet as exampled by many people on the ketogenic diet reporting they have more focus and energy running off ketones compared to other diets.

The Difference Between the Ketogenic Diet and Low Carb Diet

There is a common misconception that being on a low carbohydrate diet automatically means that your body will enter a state of ketosis. This is simply not true. To be in a state of ketosis means that the ketone reading in your blood is .5mmol/l or higher. So, even if you lower the amount of carbohydrates in your diet, it is simply not enough to put your body into a state of ketosis.

According to Health Line, the average American male adult will consume anywhere from 250 to 300 grams of carbs per day whereas a low carbohydrate diet is confirmed at 250 grams or lower per day. For most people, weight loss occurs when you lower your carbohydrate intake to 100 grams or lower. While on the ketogenic diet, as you will be learning later, it's recommended to take in 50 grams of carbohydrates or less.

On the ketogenic diet, the optimal range for ketosis is anywhere between .5 and 3.0 mmol of ketones in your blood levels. If your blood levels are under, you are not in ketosis, and if they are over, then you are either entering starvation or are at risk of ketoacidosis. This will be covered later in the book. In the following chapters, you will learn all about the risks of ketoacidosis and how to avoid it. For now, however, focus on the optimal ketone zone which you will want to keep yourself in.

The ketogenic diet is more than just restricting your carbohydrates. Yes, you can be on a low carb diet and be in ketosis, but you do not necessarily need to BE on a low-carb diet in order to be in ketosis. However, the stricter you are with your carbs, the more likely you will be able to enter this state of ketosis. What is important to realize is that it will take more than lowering your carb intake to switch your body to ketones.

Types of Ketosis

There are a couple of ways to enter ketosis besides the popular practice of lowering your carb intake and consuming foods that are higher in fat. This specific type of ketosis is known as nutritional ketosis. Below, we will outline several other ways of entering ketosis if you feel the more popular way doesn't fit your lifestyle.

Carbohydrate-Restricted Ketosis:

This is one of three variations of nutritional ketosis, and one of the most popular. As mentioned previously, this is a low carbohydrate, moderate protein, and high-fat diet. Originally, this was the standard treatment for seizures before the development of anti-epileptic drugs. Diet is very important in this version of ketosis; however, the macronutrient distribution can change drastically in individuals. When on a high fat and low carb diet, there is an increase in fat oxidation, so this diet is best for those who are looking for a sustainable, long-term approach to the ketogenic diet.

Supplemental Ketosis:

For some of the benefits that come with the ketogenic diet, it will take a bit more than restricting your carb intake for this diet to be effective. This is especially true at the levels of ketones that can be a bit difficult to maintain while on the ketogenic diet. For those who have trouble keeping their levels steady, there are supplements for this. As mentioned earlier, there are supplements known as MCTs which help you to maintain and increase ketone levels for a longer period of time. If you have chronic health issues and are attempting to cure them with a change in your diet, you will want to consider this version of the ketogenic diet.

Fasting Ketosis:

Ketosis occurs when blood glucose and insulin levels drop in your body at which point the fat oxidation begins to increase, allowing your body to produce the ketones. At first, this will only be about .1 mmol/L to .3 mmol/L. As you continue to fast, the number of ketones will increase. If you are looking for a jumpstart way to enter ketosis, this is the best option for you.

Signs You are in Ketosis

There are several symptoms that you may experience, so we suggest going to the doctor's office to officially test if you are in a state of ketosis. The tests you can take include a breath test, a blood test, and a urine test. However, if you choose to skip going to the doctor, there are several signs of ketosis you can detect by yourself. Keep a close eye out for the following signs to assure you are in a state of ketosis:

• Dry Mouth: As your body enters ketosis, you may find your mouth becoming drier than usual or that you feel thirstier. If you notice either symptom, it is very important to increase your water intake. Ultimately, you will want to be sure that you are well hydrated while on the ketogenic diet.

• Increased Urination: As you drink more liquids, you will also notice an increased need to urinate. Additionally, acetoacetate, one of the ketone bodies, are able to build up in your urine. You can take an at-home urine test to determine the number of acetoacetates in your urine.

• Ketone Scent: One of the more popular symptoms of the ketogenic diet is the ketogenic smell. For many people, this is what is known as "ketone breath", but it can also be produced via sweat. For some, this scent is fruity, but for others, it can smell like nail polish remover.

• Loss of Hunger: For those looking to lose weight, this may be an exciting symptom for you to experience. Many people on the ketogenic diet experience a reduced appetite which is mostly due to the way that the body burns energy by using fat storage while in ketosis. Some people have even reported eating one or two meals a day while on the ketogenic diet and still feeling satisfied.

• Increased Energy: It is important to realize that you may feel very tired when you first start the ketogenic diet. This is natural because, for the most part, your body has been running on carbohydrates for a long time, and now you are starting to create energy from fat! Once your body enters ketosis, you may begin to feel more energetic after a short period of being tired.

How to Measure Ketones

Measuring your ketone level is going to be vital during this diet. It is important that you keep your body in a state of ketosis so that you don't have to keep fasting to get back into it. Luckily for you, there are three fairly easy ways to measure your ketone levels which will be discussed in detail later on in the book to help you figure out which method best suits your lifestyle.

Urine Strips

For many people, this is the cheapest and easiest way to measure your ketones. If you are just beginning the ketogenic diet, this may be the best option for you as you simply have to stick the strip into a cup of your fresh urine. The strip's color will then change depending on the level of ketones that are in your system in that moment. If the strip turns a dark purple color, you will know that you are indeed in a state of ketosis.

The benefit of using urine strips is that they are available at most pharmacies. Additionally, they are also pretty reliable at indicating if your body is truly in a state of ketosis. The downfall, however, is that these results will vary depending on how much liquid you have been drinking and they are also unable to indicate the exact level of ketosis you are at, which is important to some people.

Breath Analyzer for Ketones

The breath analyzer is a device that is able to measure the amount of ketones on your breath, so this may be a good device for you to check your body's ketosis level if you are short on time. The good news is that this device is both simple and reusable, unlike urine strips; however, it may not always be reliable. This is because the number of ketones on your breath can change depending on the time of day, and may even change from breath to breath. If you do not need an exact number, this still may be a good option for you!

Blood Meter for Ketones

If you are not queasy at the sight of blood, the ketone meter blood test may be a good option for you. This is the most reliable method currently available, but the device itself tends to be fairly expensive. Additionally, if you have a low pain tolerance, this will not be a feasible option as you will need to prick your finger for each test.

Regardless of which method you choose, one of these options will be important to have while on the ketogenic diet. Now that you have an understanding of the ketogenic diet and its history, it's time to begin your journey. In the next chapter, you will learn all of the incredible benefits of the ketogenic diet including weight loss, lowered blood pressure, and cancer prevention just to name a few. Once you determine if the ketogenic diet is right for you, continue reading this book and learn how to get started on this incredible lifestyle.

Chapter 2: Keto Diet Benefits and Risks

All types of low-carb diets have been on the table of controversy for quite a few years. It has been said that diets high in fat content would raise cholesterol levels through the roof, causing heart disease, and other bad body ailments. But research has been changing the face of low-carb dieting. It has been shown that amongst other diets, those low-carb ones are the ones that seem to win the race. They are not only a great substitute when trying to lose weight, but they even have other great health benefits, even reducing cholesterol levels. Here are some ways that the Ketogenic Diet could produce some good things in your life!

Benefits of the Keto Diet

As you have learned, the basis of ketogenic dieting is centered on a diet that is low in the consumption of carbohydrates, low enough to switch your body from using glucose as energy to utilizing fat, which creates ketones that help you to maximize your health and fitness benefits.

In this chapter, you will learn about the vast array of benefits that come along with jumping on the ketogenic train that can help you to feel like a brand new, healthier human being!

Suppresses hunger and cravings

Many diets out there require you to eat less than your body is used to. This means that never-ending hunger pains are bound to strike and at the worst times. This is the main reason people tend to feel miserable while on any diet plan. Diets that are low in carb intake are great because it automatically reduces your appetite. Those who cut carbs and consume more proteins and fat actually eat fewer calories.

Better potential for losing weight

It doesn't take a scientist to know that reducing the number of carbs you eat will contribute to weight loss. People who stick within the means of low-carb diets lose weight at a much faster rate than those who are within the means of a low-carb diet. Diets low in carbohydrates tend to help in the reduction of excess water in our bodies, which can add on the pounds. The ketogenic diet reduces insulin levels too, meaning the kidneys are shedding all that excess sodium that can lead to retaining extra weight.

Better focused brain

Ketogenic diets were noted clear back in the 1920s to treat epileptic children. The precise mechanism that aided in seizure prevention still remains a mystery, but many researchers have no doubt that it has to do with the increase of stable neurons in the brain and the increased regulation of the mitochondria and enzymes that make up our brains.

Direct effects of the ketogenic diet when it comes to our mind are:

•   Better mental clarity

•   Better focus

•   Fewer occurrences and intenseness of migraines

Ability to fight cancer

The supplementation of ketones lessens the viability of tumor growth and lengthens the survival of those with metastatic cancer, as well as other cancers, which are currently being researched.

Prevents heart disease

When you keep your blood glucose levels low and stabilized, the better your entire body! The ketogenic diet helps to prevent high blood pressures and lowers triglyceride levels.

Many see the keto diet as counterintuitive when it comes to erasing the development of heart disease due to the major increase of fat, but it has been found that the consumption of excess carbs, especially fructose, is a key contributor to a high triglyceride level.

Decreases inflammation

The ketogenic diet is making giant strides in studies that are related to the negative results of inflammation in the body. It has been found to be highly anti-inflammatory and helps with a wide variety of health issues.

Thus, the keto diet helps to treat:

- Arthritis

- Eczema

- Psoriasis

- IBS

- Acne

- Pain

- And more

Improved energy levels and quality of sleep

Many beginners who undergo the ketogenic diet report that just after a few days that they have a positive increase in energy levels paired with a lack of cravings for carbs and bad fats. This is because the keto stabilizes insulin levels as well as produces a more readily available energy source that our brains and bodily tissues like better.

Improvement of sleep is still a bit of a mystery, however. The ketogenic diet has been proved to improve sleep thanks to the decrease in REM and increasing the slow-wave sleep patterns that are necessary for quality sleep. Researchers believe that the correlation is related to the biochemical shift that occurs in the brain after ketones are used for energy while other bodily tissues are busy burning fats.

Keep uric acid levels in check

If you have ever experienced kidney stones or gout, then perhaps the ketogenic diet is for you so you never have to deal with these terrible pains again! What causes these painful ailments is the increase in phosphorus, uric acid, and calcium levels in the body. This occurs thanks to not so great genetics, but mainly due to high consumptions of sugar, being overweight, being dehydrated, and eating and drinking items with alcohol and purines, such as meats and beers.

The ketogenic diet works by temporarily allowing uric acid levels to rise, especially during times of dehydration, and then come down over a period of time.

Better gastrointestinal and gallbladder health

Foods that are grain-based and/or sugary, such as nightshade veggies tend to increase your likelihood of getting heartburn and acid reflux. When you get yourself on a low carb diet, you will find that these ailments drastically improve and may even completely disappear. This is because low carb diets help to eradicate inflammation and autoimmune responses.

Assisting in women's health

Over the last decade, there has been much research to show that the ketogenic diet plays a vital role in the enhancement of fertility in women. Low carb diets eliminate symptoms such as prolonged or infrequent periods, obesity, and acne.

This is because women are better able to keep their blood sugars stabilized, which results in lower insulin levels throughout the body, allowing hormones to become stable.

Better eye health

All diabetics will inform you that their disease is detrimental to their eyesight and leads to an increase in the development of cataracts. When you keep your blood sugars low and stable, you will undoubtfully improve your eyesight over time.

Improvement in muscle gain and endurance

Low carb diets, especially the ketogenic, have been shown to promote the gain of muscle, which is why it is a go-to diet for bodybuilders. It allows people to gain more muscle and lose more fat.

Spares losing muscle while curbing metabolic syndrome, obesity, and diabetes

I am sure you have seen a number of articles that include "diabetes", "ketogenic", and "ketosis" in the title. Ketogenic dieting is very helpful for those with either type 1 or type 2 diabetes for all the reasons that have been previously talked about in this chapter.

• Therapy for some brain disorders – There are certain areas of our brains that strictly run on glucose as a fuel. This is the reason behind why our livers produce it from protein if we do not consume carbs. There are bigger portions of our brains, however, that burn through ketones. Think back to Charlie Abraham, who was mentioned earlier in this chapter. In studies, more than half of children who utilized the ketogenic diet had a 50% reduction in seizures. This diet, among other low-carb diets, is being studied as to what its effect is on brain disorders like Parkinson's and Alzheimer's disease.

Risks of the Keto Diet

Just like with every good thing in the world, there are some risk factors to consider before diving head first on your journey with the ketogenic diet.

Fatigue and irritability

Even though raised ketone levels can drastically improve a few areas regarding your physical quality of life, they are also directly related to feeling tired and having to work harder during physical activities.

"Brain Fog"

If you stay on the ketogenic diet long term, there is going to be some major shifting when it comes to the metabolic areas of the body. This can make you moody and somewhat sluggish, which can make you not able to think clearly or adequately focus. Ensure that you are reducing your levels of carb intake at steady levels, not all at once.

Lipids may fluctuate

Even though fats on the ketogenic diet are welcomed, if you consume large amounts of saturated fats, your cholesterol levels will begin to increase. Make sure you are consuming healthy fats.

Micronutrient deficiencies

Diets that consist of low-carb foods are more than likely lacking in essential nutrients, such as magnesium, potassium, and iron. You might want to strongly consider finding a high-quality multivitamin to take daily.

Development of ketoacidosis

If your ketone levels become too wacky, it may lead to this condition. pH levels within your blood decrease, creating an environment that is high in acidity, which can be threatening for those with diabetes.

Muscle loss

As you consume less energy, your body leans on the help of other tissues as a source of fuel. When working out heavily while on a diet like the ketogenic, there is the potential for major muscle loss.

Chapter 3: Basics of the Ketogenic Diet

The Ketosis Process

The word ketosis comes from the word "ketone," the process during which fats are broken in the body to produce energy and Ketones. A high level of ketosis means a greater number of ketones. In the absence of complex carbohydrates, the fats are forced to break down and produce ketones which are highly beneficial for active metabolism. To make this all happen, a special meal plan is required known as "Ketogenic diet." It describes a sum whole of all the eatables which are low in carbs and high in fats. Thus allowing the body to extract energy directly from fats and not from the glucose. The diet plan is prescribed to treat a number of diseases like diabetes, epilepsy, obesity and heart problems.

However, there are certain complexities related to this diet as, and it should always be opted with the guidance of a professional nutritionist, at least at the beginning when it is essential to learn about the basics of ketosis and the right approach to switch to a balance ketogenic diet.

What to Have on a Ketogenic Diet:

To make things simple and easier, let's break it down a little and try to understand the Keto diet plan as a chart explaining what to have and what not to have. Down below is a brief list of all the items which can be used on a Ketogenic diet.

- Meat of all types:

There is no restriction on meat for a keto diet. Whether it is poultry, beef, pork, lamb, or seafood, all kinds of meat can be freely enjoyed on a keto diet, as they don't contain any extra carbs or sugars.

- Vegetables:

Keep this in mind that not all vegetables are low on carbs. There are some who are full of starch, and they need to be avoided. A simple technique to access the suitability of the vegetables for a keto diet is to check if they are 'grown above the ground' or 'below it.' All vegetables which are grown underground are a no go for Keto whereas vegetables which are grown above are best for keto and these mainly include cauliflower, broccoli, zucchini, etc.

- Green Vegetables:

Among the vegetables, all the leafy green vegetables can be added to this diet which includes spinach, kale, parsley, cilantro, etc.

- Seeds and Dry Nuts:

Nuts and seeds like sunflower seeds, pistachios, pumpkin seeds, almonds, etc. can all be used on a ketogenic diet.

- Keto Fruits:

Not all berries are Keto friendly, only choose blackberries or raspberries, and other low carb berries. Similarly, not all fruits can be taken on a keto diet, avocado, coconut, etc. are keto friendly whereas orange, apples, and pineapple, etc. are high in carbohydrates.

- Vegetable Fats:

Following oils and fats can be used on a ketogenic diet: olive oil, coconut oil, palm oil, etc.

- Dairy Products:

Not every dairy product is allowed on a keto diet. For example, milk is a no-go for keto whereas hard cheeses, high fat cream, butter, eggs, etc. can all be used.

- Keto Sweeteners:

As sugar is strictly forbidden for a ketogenic diet, may it be brown or white there is a certain substitute which can be used like stevia, erythritol, monk fruit, and other low-carb sweeteners.

Table: Food to Have

Meat	Healthy Oils Dairy	Fruits	Vegetables	Nuts
Chicken	Almond oil	Avocados		
	Artichoke hearts	Almonds	Coconut milk	
Turkey	Avocado oil	Blueberries	Arugula	
	Brazil nuts	Almond milk		
Quail	Cacao butter	Coconuts	Asparagus	
	Hazelnuts/filberts	Coconut cream		

Duck	Coconut oil	Cranberries	Bell	peppers
	Macadamia nuts		Vegan butter	
Beef	Flaxseed oil	Lemons	Beets	Pecans
	Chooooo			
Mutton		Hazelnut oil	Limes Bok	choy
	Peanuts	Silken Tofu		
Lamb	Macadamia nut oil		Olives Broccoli	
	Pine nuts			
Pork	MCT oil	Raspberries	Brussels	
sprouts		Walnuts		
Fish	Olive oil	Strawberries	Cabbage	
	Chia			
Scallops		Healthy Oils	Tomatoes	Carrots
	Hemp			
Mussels		Almond oil	Watermelon	
	Cauliflower	Pumpkin		
Shrimp			Celery	

Foods to Avoid on a Ketogenic Diet:

Avoiding carbohydrates is the main aim of following a ketogenic diet. While most vegetarians may take following food items on a regular basis but they are considered as Keto Friendly. In fact any amount these items, drastically increased the carbohydrate value of your meal. So it is best to avoid their use completely.

Sugar:

Besides white and brown sugar there are other forms of it which are also not keto friendly, this list includes honey, agave, maple syrup, etc. Also, avoid chocolates which are high in sugar. Use special sweeteners and sugar-free chocolates only.

Legumes:

Legumes are also the underground parts of the plants. Thus, they are highly rich in carbohydrates. Make no mistake of using them in your diet. These include all sorts of beans, from Lima to chickpeas, Garbanzo, black, white, red, etc. cross all of them off your grocery list if you are about to go keto. All types of lentils are also not allowed on a keto diet.

Grains:

All types of grains are high in carbohydrates, whether its rice or corn or wheat. And product extracting out them is equally high in carbs, like cornflour, wheat flour or rice flour. So while you need to avoid these grains for keto, their flours should also be avoided. Coconut and almond flours are a good substitute for that.

Dairy:

As stated above, not all dairy products can be freely used on a ketogenic diet. Animal milk should be strictly avoided.

Fruits:

Certain fruits need to be avoided while on a keto diet. Apples, bananas, oranges, pineapple, etc. all fall into that category. Do not use them in any form. Avoid using their flesh, juice, and mash to keep your meal carb free.

Tubers:

Tubers are basically the underground vegetables, and some of them are rich in carbs including potatoes, yams, sweet potatoes, beets, etc.

Table: Food to Avoid

Sugars	Legumes Dairy	Grains	Fruits	Tubers	
White Milk	Lentils	Rice	Apples	Yams	Animal
brown	Chickpeas	Wheat	Banana		Potatoes
Maple syrup	Black beans Beets	Corn	Pineapples		
agave	Garbanzo beans	Barley	Oranges		
honey	Lima Beans	Millet	Pears		
Confectioner's sugar	Kidney beans Pomegranate	Oats			
Granulated sugar	White beans Watermelon	Quinoa			

«Frequently Asked Questions»

- How to calculate daily carb intake?

Whenever you follow a recipe, look for its contents and the nutritional value available with the recipe. If it is not available, look for online nutrition calculators which enable you to calculate the nutritional value within a few minutes.

- Do I need to count calories? Do calories matter?

Keeping track of caloric intake is important as it directly relates to weight gain. Whether on a low carb diet or on a high one, it is necessary to keep check of the calories.

- Is there any difference between a low-carbohydrate diet and a ketogenic diet?

A low carbohydrate diet is a general term used to describe any diet containing 130 to 150 grams total. However, ketogenic diets are the subset of this general diet plan. It further restricts the amount of carbohydrate to minimum levels and at the same time requires an increased intake of fat. Thus a ketogenic diet plan is more specific than the low carbohydrate plan.

- After how much time ketosis start to take place?

If you are a person of discipline and routine, then it usually takes 2 to 3 days to start a keto routine. However, it is a gradual process and goes through different stages. Exercise helps boosts the speed of the process. For people with sedentary lifestyles, it can also take weeks.

- What kind of dairy products is keto friendly?

Not all dairy products are keto friendly as raw dairy products are rich in carbohydrates. But those fermented or processed loses their carbohydrates and are good to use; these include butter, cheese, and yogurt.

- Are fruits allowed on a ketogenic vegetarian diet?

Yes, fruits with low amounts of carbohydrates, like coconut, strawberries, raspberries, avocado, etc. are allowed. This list also includes tomato, which is also a keto friendly fruit. However, fruits which are high in sugar should be avoided.

- Can I use sugars?

No, sugars are strictly forbidden on a ketogenic diet. Sugars can, however, be replaced with special sweeteners available in the markets. Using sweeteners is a tricky part of the ketogenic diet. While there many available in the market, there are few who are mostly used like stevia, erythritol, swerve, etc. These sweeteners are a good substitute for any sugar when used in the right proportion. As the sweetness of these sweeteners varies, always compare the proportions and then add them to the recipe.

- What kinds of fermented food products are allowed on a ketogenic diet?

Products like sauerkraut, plain yogurt, kombucha, kimchi, are all fermented, and they are also keto friendly. They help in better digestion and strengthen the immunity system of the body due to a large number of probiotics present in them. Their regular intake is vital for active metabolism.

- Are peanuts allowed?

Not all legumes are non-ketogenic; peanuts are one of them. There is a great misconception that peanuts can't be taken on a keto diet, but it is clearly not true as they are low on carbs and high in fats. When taken in small amounts, they do not disrupt the balance of the ketogenic diet.

• Is ketosis dangerous for human health?

There is no proven evidence which could suggest that ketosis is dangerous. Many people confuse ketosis with the ketoacidosis; the latter is a health problem which only occurs in patients with diabetes type 1. During ketoacidosis, the ketone level in the blood exceeds up to a critical value. Ketosis, on the other hand, is completely normal and doesn't pose any danger to a person's health.

• Aren't high-fat diets unhealthy? Isn't eating so much fat going to make me fat?

Most of us believe that high fats are unhealthy, but it is nothing but a myth. Fats can only be unhealthy if taken with the high amount of carbohydrates. However, when taken with low carbs or no carbs, these fats become a direct and active source of energy for the body. They easily break down and releases essential compounds including ketones.

Signs You are in Ketosis

There are several symptoms that you may experience, so we suggest going to the doctor's office to officially test if you are in a state of ketosis. The tests you can take include a breath test, a blood test, and a urine test. However, if you choose to skip going to the doctor, there are several signs of ketosis you can detect by yourself. Keep a close eye out for the following signs to assure you are in a state of ketosis:

•   Dry Mouth: As your body enters ketosis, you may find your mouth becoming drier than usual or that you feel thirstier. If you notice either symptom, it is very important to increase your water intake. Ultimately, you will want to be sure that you are well hydrated while on the ketogenic diet.

•   Increased Urination: As you drink more liquids, you will also notice an increased need to urinate. Additionally, acetoacetate, one of the ketone bodies, are able to build up in your urine. You can take an at-home urine test to determine the number of acetoacetates in your urine.

•   Ketone Scent: One of the more popular symptoms of the ketogenic diet is the ketogenic smell. For many people, this is what is known as "ketone breath", but it can also be produced via sweat. For some, this scent is fruity, but for others, it can smell like nail polish remover.

•   Loss of Hunger: For those looking to lose weight, this may be an exciting symptom for you to experience. Many people on the ketogenic diet experience a reduced appetite which is mostly due to the way that the body burns energy by using fat storage while in ketosis. Some people have even reported eating one or two meals a day while on the ketogenic diet and still feeling satisfied.

•   Increased Energy: It is important to realize that you may feel very tired when you first start the ketogenic diet. This is natural because, for the most part, your body has been running on carbohydrates for a long time, and now you are starting to create energy from fat! Once your body enters ketosis, you may begin to feel more energetic after a short period of being tired.

How to Measure Ketones

Measuring your ketone level is going to be vital during this diet. It is important that you keep your body in a state of ketosis so that you don't have to keep fasting to get back into it. Luckily for you, there are three fairly easy ways to measure your ketone levels which will be discussed in detail later on in the book to help you figure out which method best suits your lifestyle.

Urine Strips

For many people, this is the cheapest and easiest way to measure your ketones. If you are just beginning the ketogenic diet, this may be the best option for you as you simply have to stick the strip into a cup of your fresh urine. The strip's color will then change depending on the level of ketones that are in your system in that moment. If the strip turns a dark purple color, you will know that you are indeed in a state of ketosis.

The benefit of using urine strips is that they are available at most pharmacies. Additionally, they are also pretty reliable at indicating if your body is truly in a state of ketosis. The downfall, however, is that these results will vary depending on how much liquid you have been drinking and they are also unable to indicate the exact level of ketosis you are at, which is important to some people.

Breath Analyzer for Ketones

The breath analyzer is a device that is able to measure the amount of ketones on your breath, so this may be a good device for you to check your body's ketosis level if you are short on time. The good news is that this device is both simple and reusable, unlike urine strips; however, it may not always be reliable. This is because the number of ketones on your breath can change depending on the time of day, and may even change from breath to breath. If you do not need an exact number, this still may be a good option for you!

Blood Meter for Ketones

If you are not queasy at the sight of blood, the ketone meter blood test may be a good option for you. This is the most reliable method currently available, but the device itself tends to be fairly expensive. Additionally, if you have a low pain tolerance, this will not be a feasible option as you will need to prick your finger for each test.

Regardless of which method you choose, one of these options will be important to have while on the ketogenic diet. Now that you have an understanding of the ketogenic diet and its history, it's time to begin your journey. In the next chapter, you will learn all of the incredible benefits of the ketogenic diet including weight loss, lowered blood pressure, and cancer prevention just to name a few. Once you determine if the ketogenic diet is right for you, continue reading this book and learn how to get started on this incredible lifestyle.

Chapter 4: Going Keto

Rushing too fast to eat: When you are first adjusting to the keto diet, it is perfectly natural for you to be in a hurry to get to your meal as it can be easy to misjudge how much you need to eat in order to reliably remain full until your next meal or scheduled snack time. Rushing is actually going to cause you to eat more than you otherwise might; however, as it takes a fair amount of time for the signals from your stomach to reach your brain and indicate that you don't actually need a second helping to feel well and truly sated.

If you make an effort to simply chew each bite of food 10 or more times before swallowing, you will find that you naturally extend your meal times past the point where you can accurately ascertain whether or not you really have had enough. Alternately you could try setting your utensils down between each bite or simply enjoying your surroundings more as opposed to limiting your meal time so that you have no choice but to rush through it as quickly as humanly possible.

Always factor in ghrelin: Ghrelin you remember, is the primary hormone that indicates whether or not you currently feel hungry, which means that ignoring it is a good way to ensure that you lose your willpower and reach for a bag of chips before you know it. The best way to keep the ghrelin gremlin at bay is to focus that your system is always digesting something new every 4 hours or so. Everyone's internal clock is different, so the first thing you are going to want to do is to eat a small, filling meal or keto-friendly snack and then time yourself to see how long it is until you are hungry again.

Unfortunately, ghrelin is also known to spike when the body's carbohydrate reserves get too low, which means you are more likely to experience these hunger spikes in the future, even if your appetite was previously on an even keel. In these situations, you will often find that sweet fat bombs will be a ketosis saver, as they satiate the ghrelin's demand for carbohydrates with the sweetness while still being filling in a healthy fashion.

Keep yourself from feeling overly hungry: When you are hungry, not just slightly peckish, but extremely famished, it is going to be a lot more difficult for you to think rationally about the situation you are in as your body will be clamoring for you to do something about the situation ASAP. It, in turn, will ultimately make it much more difficult for you to think rationally about the situation, potentially putting your state of ketosis in jeopardy.

Luckily, it is extremely easy to prevent this scenario from occurring, all you need to do is plan ahead and have something that is keto friendly already lined up to guarantee that you never have to make a choice between the feeling of extreme hunger or sticking to the keto lifestyle. Additionally, it is important that you make a concentrated effort to never skip meals and always eat at the same time every day to make it easier for your body to know when its next meal is scheduled so it can act accordingly.

Don't completely ignore calories: While following a ketogenic lifestyle means that you don't need to worry about counting calories as much as you would with many other diets, it doesn't mean you should ignore them completely. While an item that is high in healthy fat and contains a medium amount of protein and a small number of carbohydrates might look good on paper, if it also weighs in at 1,000 calories per serving, then you are going to want to give it a wide berth no matter what. As such, it is helpful to have a general idea of the number of calories someone of your age, gender and lifestyle should try and consume in a given day and do your best to stay somewhere within the healthy zone. After all, just because you are going the extra mile to eat in a healthy fashion doesn't mean there is nothing else you can do to be more all-around healthy at all times.

Drink more water: Remember, being in a state of ketosis is going to naturally dehydrate your body more quickly than would otherwise be the case. This notion is not the only reason why you should ensure you are drinking at least a gallon of water a day if not more as doing so will also help you feel full for a prolonged period of time, a useful thing to remember if your carbohydrate cravings ever get to be too much to handle. If you are switching to the ketogenic diet especially for the lean look it can provide, then you may also be interested to note that the amount of water weight that you retain actually decreases the more hydrated you stay over a prolonged period of time.

Reduce your salt intake: While an overabundance of salt can lead to health problems, even a statistically average salt intake can still cause issues when it comes to losing weight as quickly and effectively as possible. Statistically speaking, you likely eat about half as much salt as you should each day to encourage maximum weight loss, as overeating will make it more difficult for you to lose those last few pounds. What's worse, it will also make you naturally feel hungrier than you otherwise would. A reduction in this area can lead to a noticeably slimmer face and stomach in as little as two weeks.

Follow the three color rule: While a diet that is based around the keto diet can be just as varied as many others, it is common for those who are just starting out to find a handful of foods that they like and stubbornly stick with them. As such, if you are looking for a way to broaden your keto horizons you may have luck forcing yourself to eat something green, something orange and something red with every meal. Foods in these colors are almost always the healthiest alternatives possible, which will, in turn, make it easier for you to naturally limit your caloric intake as well. What's more, foods in these hues are often known for helping you look and feel as young as possible, naturally highlighting the ketogenic diet's ability to help make you look and feel better than you have in years.

Add more spice to your meals: If you find yourself feeling full at the end of a meal and then making poor choices as a result because you feel the need to snack, then the composition of your meals might be fine when it comes to macronutrients; what you may be lacking is a little extra spice in your meal. Ingredients such as hot sauce that contain capsaicin

(Cerner Multum, Inc., 2018), a key component in making spicy foods spicy, are also known to naturally cause the body to release endorphins as a result. While endorphins are primarily known for making you happy, they also pull double duty and curtail your appetite as well.

Don't be afraid to break your schedule: While it is important to help your body to get into a regular routine when it comes to mealtime, that doesn't mean that if you miss a scheduled meal, then the best case is to simply skip it and wait for the next one. Missing a meal entirely is only going to lead to overeating eventually, which has the potential to kick you out of ketosis in the process. All said you should be sure to try and eat at least 70 percent of your daily caloric total before dinner and the rest at that point. Furthermore, you are going to want to ensure that you leave at least an hour and a half after dinner before you go to bed to maintain proper digestion.

Consider precooking: When it comes to sticking with the keto diet, it is wise to plan ahead and this means ensuring that you have the types of meals you need at the ready to ensure that you have the ability to really make good choices when it comes time to find a meal, even if you are on the go. While this might make sense in theory, in practice you are going to need to set aside a fair amount of time, and a substantial chunk of your food budget all at once, to ensure that you are able to properly finish what you intend to start. While it will require a dedicated time commitment, it won't be nearly as bad as you might think as long as you do it all at once. Not only will this make it easier to always choose the keto option, no matter what, but it will also make it easier to eat smaller portions, decrease your salt intake and more easily track the specifics, including calories when compared with rolling the dice on meals that you eat when you go out with friends.

Keep the serving dish out of your eyeliner: While it might not seem like it at the time, much of the hunger that you feel around mealtime is psychological. As such, you are much more likely to feel the need to reach for a second helping of breakfast lunch or dinner, if the means to go about doing so is within arm's length. With this in mind, you can beat your mind at its own game by simply plating your food ideally in another room, or at the very least out of your eyesight. This way your food will have more time to settle before you go back for seconds, helping you to regain control in the process.

Keep a food journal: Early on, it will likely feel that almost everywhere you turn you are coming face to face with a food that has a hidden number of carbs or not enough healthy fats to get the job done. As such, you may find it helpful to keep a food journal to help you keep track of everything you are eating, when, why and how. Not only will this tool help you to remember favorite new recipes with ease, but it will also enable you to catch yourself if the occasional off-diet snack turns into a full-blown habit. While it can be an extremely useful way to keep your diet in check, it only works if you stick with it 24 hours a day and 7 days a week. An incomplete food journal is of no good to anyone, so if you plan on not wasting your time, make a serious commitment and stick with it.

Wait out your cravings: While willpower is one powerful, there are physical activities that you can do to ensure that the effects of your current carbohydrate craving are as minimal and as brief as possible. In fact, there is a pair of yoga moves that you can do that will make it easier to quiet your thoughts and fight your cravings at the same time.

The first of these is a simple modified forward bend from a standing position. To perform this movement, you want to start by stand roughly 12 inches from a wall, facing away from it, with your feed planted at hip-width. From there, you will want to lean your back against the wall before bending your knees and folding your chest down onto your thighs. From this position, you will then want to breathe deeply between 6 and 12 times, making a special point to focus on the moments you are exhaling. When you feel the craving start to pass, you are going to want to slowly return to a leaning position. If, after 12 breaths your craving has not subsided, you will then want to return to a leaning pose and repeat the process.

The second pose that is known to help fight carbohydrate cravings is what is known as the child's pose. It helps to produce what many think of like a relaxed, introspective state, the purpose of which is to allow you to really look within and determine where the root of your current craving lies. After completing this exercise, you may realize that you weren't even hungry, to begin with.

To start, you will want to kneel on the floor while sitting on your heels. Your knees should be planted firmly at roughly hip width or whatever is comfortable. Your hands should be placed onto your thighs with your palms facing downward. Once you are in this position, you are going to want to slowly inhale and at the same time, move your chest forward, so that it connects with your thighs, ideally resting your head on the ground while doing so. With your head on the ground, you will then want to move your hands, so they are resting on either side of your legs with the palms facing upwards. You may hold this position until the craving subsides.

You now know the science behind the keto diet and why it works. In this chapter, you'll learn how to get started and maximize success. Here's a quick and easy step-by-step guide to use as you begin, and to refer to any time throughout your journey, for support and guidance.

Step 1: Clean Out Your Pantry

Out with the old, in with the new. Having tempting, unhealthy foods in your home is one of the biggest contributors to failure when starting any diet. To succeed, you need to minimize any triggers to maximize your chances. Unless you have the iron will of Arnold Schwarzenegger, you should not keep addictive foods like bread, desserts, and other non–keto friendly snacks around.

If you don't live alone, be sure to discuss and warn your housemates, whether they're significant others, family, or roommates. If some items must be kept (if they're simply not yours to throw out), try to agree on a special location to keep them out of sight. This will also help anyone you share your living space with understand that you are serious about starting your diet, and will lead to a better experience for you at home overall (people love to tempt anyone on a diet at first, but it will get old and they'll tire quickly).

STARCHES AND GRAINS

Get rid of all cereal, pasta, rice, potatoes, corn, oats, quinoa, flour, bread, bagels, wraps, rolls, and croissants.

SUGARY FOODS AND DRINKS

Get rid of all refined sugar, fountain drinks, fruit juices, milk, desserts, pastries, milk chocolate, candy bars, etc.

LEGUMES

Get rid of beans, peas, and lentils. They are dense with carbs. A 1-cup serving of beans alone contains more than three times the amount of carbs you want to consume in a day.

PROCESSED POLYUNSATURATED FATS AND OILS

Get rid of all vegetable oils and most seed oils, including sunflower, safflower, canola, soybean, grapeseed, and corn oil. Also eliminate trans fats like shortening and margarine—anything that says "hydrogenated" or "partially hydrogenated." Olive oil, extra-virgin olive oil, avocado oil, and coconut oil are the keto-friendly oils you want on hand.

FRUITS

Get rid of fruits that are high in carbs, including bananas, dates, grapes, mangos, and apples. Be sure to get rid of any dried fruits like raisins as well. Dried fruit contains as much sugar as regular fruit but more concentrated, making it easy to eat a lot of sugar in a small serving. For comparison, a cup of raisins has over 100 grams of carbs while a cup of grapes has only 15 grams of carbs.

Yes, you're "getting rid" of unwanted foods in your pantry, but these foods can feed many others. Please, don't throw them away! Find a local food bank or homeless youth shelter to donate them to.

Your pantry will seem empty after the cleanout. That's because products meant for longer-term storage are usually high in carbs and full of unhealthy additives and preservatives. You'll fill your refrigerator shortly (Step 2) with healthy, natural foods.

FINDING SUPPORT

Sticking to your diet in the beginning can prove difficult when close friends and family aren't eating the same as you. Even worse, they are eating all the things you're trying not to eat. Every person is different, and you likely know who will support you and who will not. For those who support you, explain that you're avoiding carbs (and which foods include carbs) and request politely that they not offer you anything when you're eating together.

Telling the naysayers that you've quit eating grains and sugar will usually suffice. The terms keto and low-carb will usually spark a debate or argument with certain people because they've been told their whole lives to eat carbs and low-fat products. Try to avoid using those terms when explaining your diet goals. Avoid direct debates by recommending they read about the benefits of being in ketosis and the health benefits of eating a low-carb diet.

Step 2: Go Shopping

It's time to restock your pantry, refrigerator, and freezer with delicious, keto-friendly foods that will help you lose weight, become healthy, and feel great!

THE BASICS

With these basics on hand, you'll always be ready to prepare healthy, delicious, and keto-friendly meals and snacks.

• Water, coffee, and tea

• All spices and herbs

- Sweeteners, including stevia and erythritol

- Lemon or lime juice

- Low-carb condiments like mayonnaise, mustard, pesto, and sriracha

- Broths (chicken, beef, bone)

- Pickled and fermented foods like pickles, kimchi, and sauerkraut

- Nuts and seeds, including macadamia nuts, pecans, almonds, walnuts, hazelnuts, pine nuts, flaxseed, chia seeds, and pumpkin seeds.

MEATS

Any type of meat is fine for the keto diet, including chicken, beef, lamb, pork, turkey, game, etc. It's preferable to use grass-fed and/or organic meats if they're available and possible for your budget. You can and should eat the fat on the meat and skin on the chicken.

All wild-caught fish and seafood slide into the keto diet nicely. Try to avoid farmed fish.

Go crazy with the eggs! Use organic eggs from free-range chickens, if possible.

VEGGIES

You can eat all nonstarchy veggies, including broccoli, asparagus, mushrooms, cucumbers, lettuce, onions, peppers, tomatoes, garlic (in small quantities—each clove contains about 1 gram of carbs), Brussels sprouts, zucchini, eggplant, olives, zucchini, yellow squash, and cauliflower.

Avoid all types of potatoes, yams and sweet potatoes, corn, and legumes like beans, lentils, and peas.

ABOUT THOSE SWEETENERS ...

The sweeteners may sound strange if you haven't heard of them before. They both come from natural sources and are safe to use in any quantity.

Stevia is extracted from the leaves of a plant called Stevia rebaudiana. Stevia has zero calories and contains some beneficial micronutrients like magnesium, potassium, and zinc. It's readily available in liquid or powder form online and in most supermarkets. It's much sweeter than sugar, so containers are usually very small—you won't need nearly as much.

Erythritol is a sugar alcohol that is low in calories, about 70 percent as sweet as sugar, and can be found naturally in some fruits and vegetables. Sugar alcohols are indigestible by the human body, so erythritol cannot raise your blood sugar or insulin levels. Several studies have proven it to be safe. Sugar alcohols can sometimes cause temporary digestive discomfort, but out of the few available sugar alcohols like xylitol, maltitol, and sorbitol, erythritol is considered to be the most forgiving and best for everyday use.

FRUITS

You can eat a small amount of berries every day, such as strawberries, raspberries, blackberries, and blueberries. Lemon and lime juices are great for adding flavor to your meals. Avocados are also low in carbs and full of healthy fat.

Avoid other fruits, as they're loaded with sugar. A single banana can contain around 25 grams of net carbs.

DAIRY

Eat full-fat dairy like butter, sour cream, heavy (whipping) cream, cheese, cream cheese, and unsweetened yogurt. Although not technically dairy, unsweetened almond and coconut milks are great as well.

Avoid milk and skim milk, as well as sweetened yogurt, as it contains a lot of sugar. Avoid any flavored, low-fat, or fat-free dairy products.

FATS AND OILS

Avocado oil, olive oil, butter, lard, and bacon fat are great for cooking and consuming. Avocado oil has a high smoke point (it does not burn or smoke until it reaches 520°F), which is ideal for searing meats and frying in a wok. Make sure to avoid oils labeled "blend"; they commonly contain small amounts of the healthy oil and large amounts of unhealthy oils.

Step 3: Set Up Your Kitchen

Preparing delicious recipes is one of the best parts of the keto diet, and it's quite easy if you have the right tools. The following tools will make cooking simpler and faster. Each one is worth investing in, especially for the busy cook.

FOOD SCALE

When you're trying to hit your caloric and macronutrient goals, a kitchen food scale is a necessary appliance. You can measure any solid or liquid food, and get the perfect amount every time. Used in combination with an app like MyFitnessPal, you'll have all the data you need to hit your goals sooner. Food scales can be found online for $10 to $20.

FOOD PROCESSOR

Food processors are critical to your arsenal. They are ideal for blending certain foods or processing foods together into sauces and shakes. Blenders don't cut it, powerwise, for many foods, especially tough vegetables like cauliflower.

One great food processor/blender is NutriBullet. The containers you blend in come with lids or drink spouts so you can take them to go or use them as storage. They're also easy to clean, making the whole system extremely convenient. They typically sell for about $80 online.

SPIRALIZER

Spiralizers make vegetables into noodles or ribbons within seconds. They make cooking a lot faster and easier—noodles have much more surface area and take a fraction of the time to cook. For example, a spiralizer turns a zucchini into zoodles, and with some Alfredo or marinara sauce, you can't tell you aren't eating noodles. Spiralizers cost around $30 and can be found in large retail stores and online.

ELECTRIC HAND MIXER

If you've ever had to beat an egg white by hand until you get stiff peaks, then you know just how difficult it is. Electric hand mixers save your arm muscles and massive amounts of time, especially when mixing heavy ingredients. You can find a decent one online for $10 to $20.

CAST IRON PANS

They've been used for centuries and were one of the first modern cooking devices. Cast iron skillets don't wear out and are healthier to use (no chemical treatment of any kind), retain heat very well, and can be moved between the stove and oven. They are simple to clean up—just wash them out with a scrub sponge without soap, dry them off, and then rub them with cooking oil. This prevents rust and encourages the buildup of "seasoning," a natural nonstick surface. Many cast iron pans come preseasoned, and this method preserves the coating. You can find them in many retail stores and online for $10 to $80, depending on the brand and size; Lodge is a popular brand, still made in the United States.

KNIFE SHARPENING STONE

Most of prep time is spent on cutting. You'll see your cutting speed skyrocket with a sharp knife set. It's also a pleasure to use sharp knives. Aim to sharpen your knives every week or so to keep them in good shape (professional chefs sharpen their knives before every use). Sharpening stones cost under $10 and can be ordered online.

KETO-FRIENDLY ALTERNATIVES

You'd be surprised just how many carbs are in common everyday foods. Below is a chart of common foods and their keto-friendly alternatives that you can enjoy at any time.

Note: Net carbs are the total carbs minus dietary fiber (soluble and insoluble) and sugar alcohols. Fiber and sugar alcohols are not counted toward net carbs because the human body cannot digest and break them down into glucose, so they do not spike blood sugar.

NICE-TO-HAVE EQUIPMENT

The kitchen section of any store can be a wonderland. There are so many intriguing gadgets. It's also nice (although not necessary) to have these other tools on hand if you can't resist the lure:

INSTANT COOKING THERMOMETER Cooking steak and chicken is much easier when you can easily prod the meat and find out whether it's at the level of doneness that you're shooting for. These can usually be found for $10 to $20 in most retail stores or online.

MEASURING SPOON SET Get the right amount of an ingredient quickly. These sets can go from $5 to $10 in any supermarket, store, or online.

TONGS Tongs reduce splatter when working quickly (compared to using a fork or spatula to flip something in a hot pan). It's best to get tongs with nylon heads so you don't scratch any of your pots or pans. You can get a pair online or in retail stores for $10 to $15.

Step 4: Meal Plan

Using meal plans in the beginning of your diet greatly increases your chances of success. The meal plans in part 2 of this book include meals for every part of the day, premade shopping lists, and macronutrient and calorie counts for each meal. They even account for leftovers. This will make starting out much easier and more enjoyable!

Meal plans work well because they give you goals and direction. If you know what you need to make next without thinking about it, you're less likely to give up, change your mind, and order food from your favorite takeout spot. Also, since you know what's coming next, you can look forward to it throughout the day and week.

Pay attention to the ingredients listed on the packaged products you buy. The best products have just a few ingredients with recognizable names, meaning they're made with fewer additives and preservatives.

After using the meal plans for a few weeks, you set your body up to have the right expectations for how much food you'll provide it and what type of food it will get (high in fat and protein and low in carbs). Even if you don't continue to use meal plans, you'll be familiar enough with the diet to know what you should be eating and how much.

CUSTOMIZING YOUR MEAL PLANS

Part 2 includes two weekly meal plans, which you can extend and reuse as many times as you like. You can also use the recipes from part 3 to make your own meal plans or swap out recipes in the meal plans provided.

The daily caloric goal in the meal plans is about 1700 calories, give or take 100 calories. If your caloric needs are higher or lower (don't forget to use an online keto calculator before you start), adjust accordingly with some of the ingredients in the meals by simply taking out a little or adding a bit more. Additionally, you can always use an extra tablespoon of olive oil or butter when cooking to get an extra 100 calories or so.

SHOPPING

Initially, you should look at the nutritional information provided for almost every packaged product to see if the product is low in carbs or not. Many companies love to add sugar, so be on the lookout. Over your first few weeks, you'll get to know which products are good and which are not as you look at nutritional labels.

Both of the meal plans in part 2 include shopping lists. You'll notice the quantities are not based on the quantities stores sell them in. Look for what would be closest to those amounts when buying the items. As you get more comfortable with your new diet and know the quantities you need, you'll rely less on shopping lists.

KETO QUOTIENT

All the recipes in this book are up to 6 grams of net carbs so you won't need to count the carbs when eating these recipes. Each recipe includes a Keto Quotient to make it easier to identify how high in fat it is.

Step 5: Exercise

As you start your diet and the pounds fall off, think about how to lose more weight or get healthier to feel even better. This is a great time to become more active through exercise.

Increase the amount you exercise relative to what you do now. If you don't exercise at all, start taking short walks or slow jogs, or a combination of both, for 15 minutes every other day. If you already go to the gym or lift weights, add an extra exercise or start doing cardio. It doesn't matter what level you're at, try to do a little more than you're doing now. That's all it takes to become healthier. Exercise is incremental, and every increment is a boost to weight loss and feeling better.

If you have the time, try taking a class or doing an activity that involves moving, like a step class or dancing, or start playing a sport like basketball. It doesn't have to be competitive, nor do you need to be good or have any previous experience. Such activities are an easy way to get on your feet, and you can learn a new skill in the process.

Staying fit through regular physical activity has been proven to reduce blood pressure and cholesterol levels as well as reduce risk for various heart diseases and type 2 diabetes. In combination with the keto diet, your health will improve dramatically, and so will your energy levels.

Any exercise, even if it's 15 minutes a week, is better than no exercise. Don't worry about how much you do in the beginning. Just start doing something and you'll build from there naturally.

EASY EXERCISE SEQUENCES

Here are a few easy exercise sequences if you're just starting out. Once every other day is enough in the beginning. If possible, try doing these with a friend or significant other for support and accountability. If you can't do some of them, that's absolutely all right! Simply focus on the ones you can do.

CARDIOVASCULAR ACTIVITY Any aerobic activity, like walking, running, or bicycling, for 15 to 30 minutes, twice a week or more.

STRENGTH CONDITIONING One set of exercises (for at least 10 repetitions, or it's too easy) targeting each of the major muscle groups: chest, shoulders, back, abs, and legs.

• Push-ups or assisted push-ups

• Pull-ups or chin-ups

• Crunches

• Squats

Chapter 5: Adverse Effects of the Ketogenic Diet

Although there are many incredible benefits that come with the ketogenic diet, there are some common side effects that you need to watch out for. Any diet will come with its fair share of common issues, and most of the time, they will stem from the same underlying issues. When you begin the ketogenic diet, you will want to remember that your body is used to running a certain way. In the following chapter, common issues you can expect, will be discussed along with ways to overcome them and how to make your transition as smooth as possible.

Causes for Side Effects

When you begin the ketogenic diet, it is possible that a variety of symptoms may occur. Studies have shown that these symptoms stem for three underlying causes including hypoglycemia, electrolyte and mineral deficiencies, and hypothalamic-pituitary-adrenal axis dysfunction. Please, do not be put off by these big terms because they will be broken down so that you have a full understanding of what is happening to your body and how you can prevent any side effects. When you start to adapt to your new keto lifestyle, your body will enter a state of shock simply because it has been running off sugar for all of these years. When you first adopt the ketogenic diet, remember that you are changing your body's fuel source from sugar to fat which will take some time getting used to.

Reason Number One: Hypoglycemia

One of the underlying causes of keto-adaption is due to hypoglycemia. This issue first occurs because your body is learning how to burn fat as fuel for what may be the first time. During this phase, you will most likely feel depressed, hungry, tired, irritable, dizzy, and have brain fog. It is important to realize that these side effects are common. The good news is that they go away after the first few weeks on the diet. Below, you will find a list of common side effects caused by hypoglycemia.

Side Effects of Hypoglycemia

•   Keto Flu: The keto flu is one of the most common side effects, and it is exactly what it sounds like. The keto flu carries many flu-like symptoms and usually happens right when you start the diet. Other symptoms that come with this flu are headaches, nausea, runny nose, and even fatigue. The good news is that this issue can be easily corrected which will be covered at the end of the chapter.

•   Sugar Cravings: A common side effect of the ketogenic diet is that people experience intense food cravings that are high in sugar. The reason the cravings may happen is because your brain enters a sort of panic mode when you first switch your diet. During this panic mode, your brain feels that you need energy from sugar or you will die. These will subside once your body begins to produce ketones as energy. As soon as this energy switch happens, your brain and body will get over thinking you're close to death.

•   Drowsiness and Dizziness: Before your body becomes fully adapted to the keto diet, you may experience drowsiness or dizziness. Luckily, this is a pretty short-term effect of the keto-adaption process and you will most likely feel this way because of a lack of energy. This is especially true if your blood pressure is dysregulated on your new diet. There are simple ways to fix this issue as we will be going over shortly.

•   Reduced Physical Performance and Strength: As you begin the ketogenic diet, your body is learning how to use a new fuel source: fat. At this point, your muscles and brain are using mitochondria as its energy production. As you switch over your diet, your body will need to learn how to use ketones. During this switch, you may experience a drop in your physical ability and strength. This is a very short-term effect but can be difficult for athletic people to endure for even a short period of time.

Strategies for Overcoming Hypoglycemia

Eat: When starting your new diet, eating properly is going to be important. It is essential to eat every three to four hours. By doing this, you will keep the hunger pangs down and your blood sugar balanced.

Drink: Along with drinking lots of water, try to drink beverages rich in minerals. This is extremely important, especially in-between meals. We suggest electrolyte drinks or even broths.

Magnesium Supplements: You may want to consider taking a magnesium supplement if you experience any side effects. By taking a supplement such as L-threonate three times a day, you may be able to reduce or lesson some of the symptoms you are experiencing.

Mineral Rich Foods: While on the ketogenic diet, you will want to use salt generously. It's also important to consume foods that are rich in minerals and that are also hydrating such as cucumbers or celery. Later on, you will learn about some of the foods that will keep you healthy on the ketogenic diet.

Exogenous Ketones: This is one of the best ways to train your body on how to use ketones. The exogenous ketones arc able to buffer any hypoglycemic effects that you may be experiencing so that your body will be able to use these ketones as energy.

Reason Number Two: HPA Axis Dysfunction

Your HPA Axis consists of three different glands including your Adrenals, Pituitary Gland, and the Hypothalamus. Together, these glands are in charge of regulating the stress response in your body. As mentioned previously, the ketogenic diet will essentially put your body into panic mode because it will think you are starving, and thus dying. In response, the adrenals will begin to release cortisol which acts as a signal to release any glucose you have stored in your body to provide you with energy. When this happens, the stores of glycogen are burned quickly, and the cycle continues.

So, what happens when this energy source is taken away? Below, you will find some of the issues caused from HPA Axis Dysfunction.

Side Effects of HPA Axis Dysfunction

Sleep Issues

One of the most common side effects caused by HPA Axis Dysfunction is sleep disruption. Due to the cortisol levels in your body, these levels will begin to fluctuate and could potentially interfere with the release of melatonin in your body. The result of this happening in your system is poor sleep quality and insomnia. The main issue is that this cortisol response is extremely helpful in emergency situations, even if your body isn't aware that there is food readily available in the fridge or at the restaurant down the road. When you are aware of what is causing your issues, it will be easier to combat insomnia.

Heart Palpitations

Another side effect that people notice when beginning the ketogenic diet is heart palpitations. This can mostly be attributed to the HPA axis dysfunction and the mineral imbalances in your body. If you are experiencing heart palpitations, this is due to the abnormally high levels of cortisol in your body. When these levels are too high for too long, your body starts to build a resistance to cortisol. So, to compensate for this, your body will start to secrete more adrenaline and as the adrenaline spikes in your body, an irregular heart rhythm is created.

Strategies for Supporting your HPA Axis

•   Magnesium Supplements: A magnesium supplement will help to support your HPA axis, which is the root of all the issues covered in this chapter. L-threonate, a magnesium supplement, has been proven to cross the blood-brain barrier which will help with both your pituitary glands and your hypothalamus.

•   Balance Blood Sugar: Taking a magnesium supplement will also help with your hypoglycemia. By balancing your blood sugar levels, you may be able to prevent the side effects of the HPA Axis dysfunction.

•   Adaptogenic Herbs: If you have tried the two strategies mentioned above to no avail, consider using some adaptogenic herbs. Studies have shown that these herbs can help you to build resilience to stress. When you are able to regulate your cortisol levels, you can avoid the side effects from the dysfunction of the HPA Axis.

Reason Number Three: Mineral and Electrolyte Deficiency

Minerals and electrolytes play a vital role in regulating your body's hydration which is very important for proper nerve conductivity. When you first enter keto-adaption, most of these minerals will be excreted through your urine thanks to your HPA axis dysregulation. As you can tell, all of these side effects are intertwined. In addition to the cortisol levels in your body, the HPA axis is also in charge of regulating the excretion and retention of the minerals in your body. When the HPA axis is dysregulated, it is easy to become dehydrated. Unfortunately, there are a number of side effects that manifest from this imbalance.

Side Effects of Mineral and Electrolyte Deficiency

Urination

One of the most obvious signs that you have a mineral and electrolyte deficiency is more frequent urination. When you begin a low-carb diet such as the ketogenic diet, your insulin levels will begin to drop. Once this happens, you will begin to secrete more sodium through your urine. This is a normal side effect of the ketogenic diet and actually is a positive sign that you are in keto-adaption.

Constipation

If you are suffering from constipation, this is most likely because you are not maintaining a proper balance of electrolytes or minerals. The ability to pass stool is influenced by water content in your body. As you make drastic changes to your diet, the microbiome will also change your stools. This is something you will want to pay special attention to when you switch over to the ketogenic diet.

Diarrhea

Conversely, some people also report experiencing diarrhea when they first start the ketogenic diet. Although constipation is more common, this may happen due to the changing microbiome in your body. If you begin to experience diarrhea on a daily basis, try activated charcoal as a binding agent to help.

Due to its strong absorption properties, activated charcoal may help to treat diarrhea by trapping bacteria and impurities in its surface. In a 2017 review published in the Journal of Current Medical

Research and Opinion, the researchers noted that it may be a suitable diarrhea treatment by protecting against bacteria and drugs from being absorbed into the body. Another benefit is that it has few side effects compared to many antidiarrheal medications.

Muscle Cramping

With poor hydration and mineral imbalance, you may begin to experience muscle cramps. Muscle cramps occur when you have an imbalance in proper nerve impulse conductivity. So, if you experience frequent muscle cramps, this may be because of a mineral imbalance within your body.

Strategies for Maintaining Proper Mineral Balances and Hydration

•   Stay Hydrated: Many of these side effects stem from being dehydrated. When you are on the ketogenic diet, be sure to stay hydrated throughout the day by drinking a lot of water, drinks with electrolytes, and even mineral-rich broths to help release toxins from your body.

•   Mineral Rich Foods: If you experience side effects such as muscle cramps and constipation, remember how important your diet is. Ensure that you are consuming mineral-rich foods such as seaweed, cucumbers, leafy greens, and celery as these are all ketogenic friendly foods and great for your health.

• Salt Quality: While on the ketogenic diet, the quality of salt in your diet is going to be very important. So, it's recommended that you use a high-quality salt, as this will add in the sodium and trace minerals you need in your diet. We recommend using Celtic Sea Salt or Pink Himalayan Sea Salt because they are both high in trace minerals.

Ketoacidosis

Ketoacidosis is one of the more serious complications of the ketogenic diet and is something that should be taken very seriously. Ketoacidosis refers to diabetic ketoacidosis, or DKA., and is caused by a complication of Type-one diabetes mellitus. This is a life-threatening condition that occurs when you have high levels of blood sugar and ketones. When this happens, the blood in your body becomes too acidic to function properly. For some people, this issue can occur in as little as twenty-four hours, particularly those who already have Type-one diabetes. Ketoacidosis symptoms to watch out for include:

- Confusion

- Shortness of Breath

- Fruity Breath Scent

- Tiredness

- Stomach Pain

- Vomiting

- Nausea

- Dehydration

- Frequent Urination

- Extreme Thirst

Causes of Ketoacidosis

One of the main causes of ketoacidosis is poor diabetes management. For example, you could suffer from DKA even if you miss even one insulin dose or if you get an infection or illness. Additionally, certain drugs can prevent your body from using insulin the way it is meant to be. Other factors include alcohol, stress, heart attack(s), or malnutrition.

Diagnosis Ketoacidosis

1.   Urine Ketone Levels: >5mmol/L

2.   Blood Ketone Levels: 1.5-3.0 + 3 mmol/L

Treatment for Ketoacidosis

If you feel that you are at risk for Ketoacidosis, seek emergency help immediately. Generally, treatment will involve screening for an infection which can be taken through fluids via mouth or vein. As a result, your doctor will most likely suggest a replacement of electrolytes, and perhaps even intravenous insulin until you can balance your blood sugar level. Regardless, you will need to seek professional help, and above all, please do not take it upon yourself to treat ketoacidosis.

Pros and Cons of the Ketogenic Diet

Neurological Benefits:

•   Epilepsy Reduction in Children

•   Cognitive and Behavioral Improvements

•   Improved Bipolar Symptoms

- Protection Against Traumatic Brain Injury

- Autism Improvements

- Neurodegenerative Disorder Improvements

Neurological Adverse Reactions:

- Impaired Mood

- Impaired Concentration

Musculoskeletal Benefits:

- Improved Athletic Performance

Musculoskeletal Adverse Reactions:

- Osteopenia

- Skeletal Fractures

- Muscle Cramps

- Muscle Weakness

Reproductive and Endocrine Benefits

- Improved Glycemic Control

- PCOS

- Increased Fat Loss

- Appetite Suppression

Reproductive and Endocrine Adverse Effects:

- Decreased Height and Weight Growth in Children

- Acute Pancreatitis

- Thinning Hair

- Hypoglycemia

- Irregular Menstruation

Cardiovascular Benefits:

- Improved Blood Lipids

Cardiovascular Adverse Effects:

- Myocardial Infarction

- Heart Arrhythmia

- Cardiomyopathy

- Hypertriglyceridemia

Ultimately, while there are some incredible benefits with this diet, there will also be some bumps along the way to changing your body for the better. If you experience any of these side effects, please consult with your doctor to ensure that they aren't more serious.

Chapter 6: Ketogenic Diet Tips and Tricks

Diets can be tough - it is totally understandable! Starting the ketogenic diet can seem overwhelming between counting your macros and having a limited diet, but remember all of the incredible benefits that come with the change. You have been provided with a complete grocery list as well as a sample meal plan to help you get started, now, it is time to learn some tips and tricks to make the diet even easier!

No Cheating!

Unlike other diets, the ketogenic diet is not one you can slip up on occasionally and not suffer the consequences. Even the slightest cheat can throw off the balance of your body trying to get into ketosis. When you feel tempted to have that brownie after dinner, think of all the hard work you are putting into your diet and tell yourself that it is not worth it. Instead, have a healthy fat-loaded snack to satisfy that craving.

Try Fermented Foods

Fermented foods can help keep away any constipation you may have while on the ketogenic diet. It is also important to stay hydrated during your new diet, so some foods you can try include kefir, coconut water, kimchi, sauerkraut, and even pickles!

Get up and Move

As you know, when you first start the ketogenic diet, you may feel very low energy. As your body gets adjusted, try to add some exercise to your routine. At first, try light exercises, but soon short, high-intensity workouts will be best, especially if you are trying to lose weight. If you need an example exercise program to get you started, try this one:

• Sunday: Upper Body + Cardio for Twenty Minutes

• Monday: Lower Body + Cardio for Twenty Minutes

• Tuesday: Recreational Activity i.e. Walking

• Wednesday: Upper Body + Cardio for Twenty Minutes

• Thursday: Lower Body + Cardio for Twenty Minutes

• Friday: Cardio for Thirty Minutes

• Saturday: Cardio, Yoga, or Rest

Stay Hydrated

Staying hydrated is going to be vital while on the ketogenic diet because you will be losing a lot of water. You will want to try your best to drink a gallon of water a day along with other helpful beverages. Please refer to the grocery list above to get some ideas of drinks that you can use to stay hydrated!

Know Healthy Carbs

While carbs are going to be very limited on the ketogenic diet, it is important to learn the difference between "good" and "bad" carbohydrates. When you know the good carbs, you will be able to get the proper nutrients you need for your diet. Try some carbs like cucumbers, asparagus, lettuce, peppers, broccoli, green beans, and spinach!

Avoid Alcohol

When it comes to dieting, you will want to think of your diet as "spending." When it comes to drinking, you have a very limited amount of carbohydrates so you will not want to waste your carb allowance on alcohol. If you do want a drink, try to stick to hard liquors, since they often have less carbs.

Fat Bombs

Do yourself a solid and learn a few fat bomb recipes as these are perfect when you are craving some sweetness and also need to boost your fat intake. These little treats are a win-win situation!

Prepare

One way that you can ensure that you stick to your new ketogenic diet is by meal prepping. When you plan everything ahead, you leave yourself very little room for failure. Take a day of the week, hit up the grocery store, and cook your meals for the week. By knowing what you are eating in advance, this leaves no room for the temptation to go through the drive-thru when you can't decide what you want to eat!

Watch the Protein

As mentioned previously, fat is the most important aspect of the ketogenic diet. While protein is going to be important as well, it is also important to know that if you eat too much protein, your body can convert it into glucose. As a general rule, stick to 1g of protein for every two pounds of body weight; this number can fluctuate depending on the activity level you are at.

Technology

Diets today can be kept track of like never before. Using your phone or some other Smart device, find an application that lets you keep a list or food diary of what you eat every day. This will be vital for keeping track of your macros through the day. You will want to create a habit of keeping track to make dieting even easier for you.

YES, you CAN

On the ketogenic diet, it can be very easy to focus on what you can and cannot eat. Instead of getting upset about the foods you are "missing out on," try changing your mindset. There are plenty of delicious foods you still can eat on this diet. It may take some extra work, but it will be worth it at the end of the day.

Diet Gimmicks

Unfortunately, diet culture has taken over grocery stores. When you are grocery shopping, avoid foods that say words like "sugar-free," "low-fat," or "light." Often times, these foods have a crazy amount of added ingredients to add flavor or are filled with carbs, which as you know, you will need to avoid!

Keep it Simple

There is absolutely no reason to get crazy and wild with your ketogenic diet. If you try to make it complicated, you will most likely sabotage your own efforts. You have been provided with a basic list to help you navigate the grocery store. Take a look at the foods you can eat along with some of the spices, and keep your recipes super simple.

Temptation Elimination

You are in charge of what is in your fridge and your cabinets. Be sure to remove any temptations you may have in your home. It's inevitable that the cravings are going to hit you when you first start the ketogenic diet, so by not having any "bad" items in your house, there will be nothing to cheat on your diet with!

Fasting

One of the best ways to get yourself into ketosis is by fasting. If you can, try to go low-carb for two or three days before you fast so that you can avoid a hypoglycemic episode. If you refer back to chapter three, you can remind yourself about the side effects that come with it. As you fast, remember to stay hydrated. Try one of the following:

- Simple Fast: 12 hours

- Cycle Fast: 16 hours - 3 times a week

- Strong Fast: 16 - 18 Hours a Day

- Warrior Fast: 19 - 21 Hours a Day

- One Day Fast: One Day - Once a Week

Utilize MCT Oil

MCT Oil is going to be beneficial when you are on the ketogenic diet. It is vital if you are looking to get into ketosis as well as maintaining it. When you consume more MCT oil, it will help you consume more carbohydrates and protein while still maintaining ketosis. The good news is that the body is able to metabolize MCT oil immediately. This is great for fast energy in your body. MCT oil is also great to add to just about anything including your coffee, drinks, shakes, and anything that you cook.

Keep Calm

If you are stressed out all of the time, this could ruin your ability to stay in ketosis. If you are going through a troubled period in your life, the ketogenic diet may not be the right diet for you in that moment. As you know, stress can raise your stress hormones which drive up your blood sugar. When this happens, it lowers the ketones in your body. Try taking up practices such as meditation or yoga to help bring peace and calmness into your life.

Listen to Your Body

You are starting a new diet, so you are more than likely going to be hungry! Now that you are on a low-carb diet, it will be important to fuel your body. When you become hungry, that is a sign that your metabolism is slowing down. If you ignore these feelings, all of your hard work will backfire at you. Keep snacks at hand to keep yourself fueled.

Bullet Proof Coffee

Looking for another way to get your fat percentage in? Try Bullet Proof coffee! This is a cup of coffee with MCT oil, unsalted butter, water, stevia, and heavy cream. This wonderful treat is high in fat content and low in carbs!

Mid-night Snacks

While on the ketogenic diet, you may get cravings right before bed. One of the best ways to get rid of these cravings is to have a piece of cheese or a cube of butter, followed by a full glass of water. For the most part, this is a good way to take care of your cravings while still staying within your diet limits! However, it's best to avoid eating late night meals before bedtime.

Weight loss strategies

Tips to stay to your fitness arrange

If losing weight was at the forefront of your mind at the beginning of the year, likelihood is that you've have already toughened some challenges by currently. Truth is, protrusive to a strict calorie controlled diet isn't straightforward for the bulk of individuals attempting to lose weight. But, maintaining a healthy diet and way is that the best strategy for weight loss. it'll conjointly improve your overall health in addition as cut back your risk of diseases.

A number of studies have shown that being attentive to calorie intakes is very important once it involves slimming down, primarily as a result of even short periods of accidental gula will cause weight gain or hinder your ability to induce obviate that stubborn belly fat. Hence, understanding however straightforward it's to engorge will facilitate with weight loss because it will assist you to be a lot of attentive to dietary selections. Here area unit 5 straightforward ways that to assist you eat healthy, follow your weight loss arrange and slem down your waist in one week.

Keep junk out of sight

The saying 'out of sight, out of mind' undoubtedly applies here - you're a lot of probably to eat unhealthy food once encircled by junk and processed foods. certify that those unhealthy food things area unit out of the house to extend the chances of reaching your weight loss goals.

Practice conscious intake

Studies have shown that adopting a conscious intake habit will increase your possibilities of constructing healthy, lasting behavioral changes. Take time to relish what you eat and appreciate its ability to nourish you. it'll improve your relationship with food and will even facilitate stop binge intake.

Set realistic goals

While that specialize in nutritive foods has several health advantages, your weight loss goals could backfire if you are trying to slenderize too quickly. analysis shows that fat those who expect to lose a great deal of weight area unit a lot of probably to drop out of a weight loss programme. Set realistic plans to extend your possibilities of staying on target.

Flexibility is that the key to success

It is probably that you'll want an explicit degree of flexibility notwithstanding that diet approach you decide - since most diets would force some compromise. All it takes is being a lot of aware of food selections within the days before or once a big day, perhaps, you'll be able to increase your exercise levels to counter any excesses.

Don't forget to exercise

Remember, diet and exercise go hand in hand particularly if your goal is to slenderize. analysis has shown that creating each dietary and physical activity changes at an equivalent time can assist you see nice results. you can't expect to realize your fitness goals quick by doing one and ignoring the opposite - it's as straightforward as that!

Easy ways in which to kick start your weight loss journey and flatten your belly while not touching the athletic facility

If you're serious regarding slimming down and ever-changing the means your body appearance, then you almost certainly apprehend the drill! ingestion a healthy diet and obtaining regular exercise will assist you shed those further kilos with success. however with numerous high-calorie health foods being simply on the market, you tend to savours binge ingestion, sabotaging your weight loss efforts. Perhaps, food portion sizes ar spinning out of management, one major reason you're pilling on the pounds.

If you're troubled to keep up a healthy diet or persist with your fitness goals, this 3-step arrange will assist you thin with marginal efforts. This strategy is straightforward, straightforward to adopt and doesn't need shopping for all varieties of completely different foods and ingredients, in contrast to most fat diets that are dear and wish following sophisticated recipes. The arrange made public here can improve your metabolism and cut back your belly fat quickly while not hunger - in as very little time as seven days.

The step arrange for fast and healthy weight loss

Step 1: This part starts you out on your thanks to healthy weight loss by limiting the intake of starchy carbohydrates. the first step encourages dieters to extend their intake of high-quality supermolecule, vegetables and healthy fats needed for effective fat burning.

Step 2: In step 2, dieters could introduce fruit and increase their intake of starchy carbohydrates. you'd need to want wholegrain types of starchy foods that are sensible sources of fibre that is required permanently organic process health and is coupled to improved weight loss. this can be thought of the transition part because it permits your body to re-adjust to manufacturing the proper quantity of hypoglycemic agent necessary whereas additionally serving to you retain the load off.

Step 3: By currently, you've learned to eat healthy and achieved your weight loss goals by creating healthier food selections and ingestion a well-balanced diet. you'll still get pleasure from your diet the means you've been tutored to keep up your weight.

Lose Weight: 5 Rules Drew Barrymore Followed To Lose Weight

I've been operating with player Barrymore for over eight years currently, and he or she is thus beloved for her realism. She is one in every of us—not good, not feeding utterly all the time—but she will perceive sure principles I even have educated her. Recently, she created headlines for her twenty five pound weight loss, that she achieved not by performing some insane diet, however by alimental her body, and her gut.

I don't assume we have a tendency to were designed to feel disadvantaged all the time. I do assume that we'd like some sweats and carbs in our life—otherwise "sweet" would not be thought-about a primary Ayurvedic style. Our brains would like some carbs to perform. i really believe life, and food, square measure meant to feel swarming, joyful, and additional packed with ease than we've typically been educated.

I teach my readers and shoppers a way of life based mostly around feeling smart. Feeling smart does not imply we have a tendency to square measure essentially happy and elated all the time; rather, it suggests that we have a tendency to square measure connected to ourselves, our bodies, and our own inner knowledge and intuition. we are able to higher comprehend what foods and decisions serve North American country, once we square measure hungry, and once we don't seem to be. we've a bigger sense of peace in our utterly imperfect lives, that is strictly what my new book (out next week), Recipes for Your utterly Imperfect Life, teaches.

With that in mind, here square measure 5 key principles I created in Drew's program to assist her, yes, lose weight and appearance nice, but, additional significantly, heal her gut and feel wonderful too.

1. very (and I mean really) nourish your gut.

If we do not have balanced guts, it suggests that our digestion is compromised, and that we tend to "hold" additional, creating weight loss abundant more durable. i spotted this years agone after I went out packing and learning for 3 years round the world, got out of the restrictions of the Western mentality, and eventually understood the affiliation of wholeness, together with between my constipation, digestion problems, and bloating and my inability to drop weight. Gut health has been stylish recently, however I've really been talking regarding this affiliation since my 1st book! you'll nourish your gut by reducing refined sugars, operation difficult-to-digest foods, like farm and protein, meditating and/or transferral in heedfulness practices to assist you handle stress (this is as vital as what you eat, in my opinion, as everything affects everything else), and taking probiotics.

2. Eat countless ginger...and different strategic foods.

Why ginger? It warms your body and will increase circulation and metabolism. It really promotes a heat feeling in your body. This helps you drop into your body and out of your head, serving to interrupt the cycle of negative circular thought patterns and anxiety. attempt creating ginger tea or adding to a soup or stir-fry after you end up turbinate into a food desire or binge cycle.

Weight loss/balance could be a semipermanent mode that's very created with reconciliation emotional, mental, and religious well-being furthermore. If we have a tendency to square measure stressed and "holding on" in our mind, manifesting as anxiety, insomnia, chronic resentments, and perpetually beating ourselves up and feeling guilty, then i think that interprets to a additional arduous time of our bodies rental go of weight. each single a part of our life flows and connects to all or any the opposite elements.

3. Drink the Glowing inexperienced Smoothie (GGS) each morning.

Our bodies would like natural foods to perform at their best, and let weight balance and lodge in a balanced level, and this includes increasing natural fullness (feeling calm around food generally versus stressed regarding it!) and digestion. This smoothie is essential therein it provides you fiber, plenty of vitamins, minerals, antioxidants and additional. you'll build it by combining seven cups cut spinach (about a medium bunch), vi cups cut cos lettuce lettuce (about one little head), two cups cold filtered water, 1½ cups cut celery (about two medium stalks), one medium apple, cored and coarsely cut, one medium pear, cored and coarsely cut, one medium banana, unclothed and cut in thirds, two tablespoons freshly squeezed juice and a few parsley and cilantro (optional), and mixing till sleek. This serves four, thus share with an admirer or save for later!

4. Avoid farm.

Across the board, I realize that the majority people's bodies open up additional and unharness once then they shift from farm to plant-based milks, cheeses, yogurts, and so on. In my observe, I've found farm to be terribly mucus-forming and symptom, thus if your goal is to lose weight and reduce, it's not a awfully useful food therein regard, as we have a tendency to try to make additional of a natural flow in your body.

5. observe current cleansing.

It's very vital we have a tendency to square measure body process (yes, I'm talking regarding gut movements!) the maximum amount as potential. Our bodies square measure competitive with endogenous (normal cell breakdown matter) and exogenous (from pollution, significant metals, environmental pollutants, and then on) toxins every and each day. The additional economical we have a tendency to square measure at cathartic, the more room there's within the body for element and nutrients to flow into.

Some measures for cleansing square measure to eat countless fiber to cleanse your system, adding cilantro to your diet to assist bind to and cleanse significant metals, avoiding refined sugars (which have a "sticky" impact on our systems), and feeding additional energy-efficient, plant-based meals.

Chapter 7: Adapting A Ketogenic Diet For Maintenance.

If you're looking at the ketogenic diet as a short term weight loss solution, simply taking on board the essentials and avoiding carbs is more than enough. However if you are chasing all-round health, you will need to be more careful with your diet.

All restrictive diets can be risky in that we are used to getting our nutrients from specific places. When we remove one or more of those foods, we can end up becoming deficient in vital nutrients. For instance, many of us get most of our dietary fibre from grains and legumes. If we cut out grains and legumes but do not eat enough nuts, seeds, and greens to increase our fibre intake, we may become deficient. Or we may get all our vitamin C from sweet fruits, so unless we start eating dark green vegetables and nonsweet fruit daily, we could accidentally run out of vitamin C.

Likewise, we are used to only eating a small amount of certain nutrients, but when we change our diet we may eat too many of them. For instance, ketogenic diets are not supposed to be very high protein, and some people are vulnerable to excess protein in their diets. And yet, when we try and increase our fat intake to promote ketosis, sometimes we will eat far, far more protein than we need. Or take vitamin A. Too much of it is poisonous, but if we decide to eat loads of liver pate, because we aren't keen on other types of offal, we could give ourselves vitamin A poisoning.

Therefore, if we are considering following a ketogenic diet long term, we need to be much more careful about the balance than if we were eating it for a week or three. We need to give careful thought to everything that enters our mouths, and ensure we eat a variety of natural, whole foods. In essence, although we are changing our macronutrient balance, by cutting carbs right down and increasing fat intake, we don't want our micronutrients to change at all, or if they do change we want to change them for the better.

There are four keys to following a ketogenic diet successfully and healthily in the long term:

1: Choosing healthy fats.

2: Eating a varied diet full of micronutrients.

3: Not neglecting fibre intake.

4: Following the 80/20 rule.

If these key factors are not approached properly, we risk losing too much weight, gaining weight, provoking inflammation, or causing malnutrition. But if we adopt all four keys to a good, healthy ketogenic diet, we will be fitter and healthier than ever before. Over the next chapters we will explore what each of those points means, and how it applies to our own personal circumstances and specific dietary needs.

Choosing healthy fats is a very important step. Many of us have been made to think of fats as unhealthy due to a misunderstanding which happened in the 1970s. When the government issued health warnings against fat, and in particular animal fats, there were hardly any cases of young people with heart disease, strokes, cancer, or obesity. These concerns had been rising very, very slightly for decades, but were still very rare. And soon after that, these health problems began to spike. Following the recommendation to eat less fat did not work. In the 90s our health issues began to taper off as we realized that olive oil is not bad for us. And now we are exploring animal fats as healthy again, beginning with the omega oils in fish, complex saturated fat in cheese, and cholesterol in eggs.

So why the sudden turn around? Well, obviously in the 70s we were wrong. The biggest factors damaging our health in those days were alcohol consumption and sugar consumption, which were both at levels never seen in any people since the aristocracy in the 1700s. We have already seen what simple sugars can do to our bodies when we eat too much of them, and how they can lead to inflammation, obesity, diabetes, etc. But the element of alcohol made things far, far worse.

Alcohol is a form of calories that is very difficult to access, as the liver needs to break it down to access the sugars. The liver has a limited amount of toxic products it can break down in a day, and just a few units of alcohol can take up all of that allowance. What does this mean in real terms? It means that when we drink, we are giving our livers too much to do, and then they start to fall behind on the rest of their work. Being drunk and having a hangover are signs that your liver is failing to do its job, signs that your body is overwhelmed with toxins.

If we overwhelm our livers and flood our bodies with toxins, our immune system needs to fight twice as hard to keep us fit and healthy. So now, until our liver is better, our immune system is working overtime as well. And when our immune system works overtime, we suffer inflammation, are at an increased risk of cancer, gain weight both in water and fat, and generally find our health declining.

Finally, alcohol consumption leads to decreased inhibitions, which in most people leads to increased food consumption, and being more likely to eat foods which we know are bad for us. Or, in other words, when we're drunk we're most likely to order a large burger meal or a kebab. We want greasy, carby, processed foods and we want it immediately. Not only do we eat worse things, but we eat things with more calories, which will naturally result in weight gain, increasing our risks of heart disease, diabetes, and strokes.

By ignoring how many simple carbs people were eating and taking the focus away from alcohol, the governmental guidelines had inadvertently promoted, not stopped, the rising health problems we were facing.

That's not to say they were entirely wrong. The fats people were eating had increased, of course, but not as part of a conscious decision, rather as vegetable oils began to form part of our processed food options. Vegetable oils are very much a misnomer, as they aren't made of vegetables, but seeds, and most commonly canola seed. There are major problems with these oils, but two stand out above all others: the quantity, and the processing. There is no way that any point in our existence we would have managed to eat four or five tablespoons of seed oil a day. That would have meant eating 50 grams of seeds every day, which would have taken most of our day to collect and press. Other fats were abundant, but these were rare. And furthermore, vegetable oils are highly processed. When fats are heated too much and hydrogenated they become oxidation-causing toxins. And almost every vegetable oil is highly processed. We will discuss the exceptions shortly.

Dietary cholesterol, which had been blamed for raised blood cholesterol, turned out to not increase your cholesterol in the long term. In the short term the cholesterol in egg yolks raises your blood cholesterol, the same way a bite of fruit raises your blood sugar. It's temporary, because what's in your stomach needs to get out. But that doesn't mean it's going to stay up. In fact, in the long term it actively reduces total blood cholesterol, triglycerides, and bad cholesterol, whilst increasing good cholesterol. The more cholesterol you eat from eggs, natural meats, and dairy, the better your blood cholesterol will get.

Saturated fat was then blamed for high cholesterol, in part thanks to a very cherry picked piece of research called The China Study, which sought to uphold the animal fat myth, so as to promote a vegetarian diet for social and political reasons. The China Study looked into traditional diets around the world, and reported that people who traditionally ate more animal fat were less healthy. How did they reach this conclusion? By removing information from countries where animal fat intake was high and health was also high. Or, the short form: vegan activists were happy that we were not eating much animal fat, and didn't want us to see that animal fat is perfectly healthy. Shockingly, it took a while before other major researchers found out about the fraud, and in that time it became such popular knowledge that it is still mentioned by activist documentaries and health gurus today. But as a fact, it has more in common with old wives tales than science. Real data shows natural saturated fat is just another healthy source of calories for the human body.

Some health food advocates would say that this means we must eat animal fats, and not plant fats, but the distinctions of quality must be made. Not all plant fats are bad for us, only the processed ones are. In fact, fats from fatty fruits and nuts are things we would have had good access to twice a year at least. This is because fatty fruit trees, like avocado and olive trees, and nut trees like walnut and brazil trees, fruit prolifically twice a year, giving us fairly easy-to access fats from their fruit. We would also have had regular access to whole seeds in the fruits we were eating. We would not have eaten much in the way of seeds, but they would have not been wasted. We would also have nibbled on some herb and grass seeds, but only in very small amounts. Pumpkin, apricot, and flax seed are all examples of seeds which we may have eaten up to a tablespoon a day of. These fats are not only natural, but are whole, unprocessed, and full of vital vitamins and minerals which will nourish our bodies. And if you want to choose an oil derived from vegetable fats, look at olive oil for cold uses and coconut oil for high temperature cooking. Olive oil is one of the healthiest plant fats around, but denatures quickly when heated. And coconut oil is a healthy plant-based saturated fat which resists high temperatures well.

Likewise, not all animal fats are good for us, only the unprocessed ones are. In the wild, healthy animals go through periods of gaining fat and periods of burning it. This means their body fat will cycle and be fairly low in toxins. They also exercise and eat natural diets. Cows eat grass and herbs; chickens eat insects and leaves and the odd bit of seed; pigs eat greens, roots, insects, and carrion, etc. You may have noticed how none of those animals naturally eat corn or wheat, two of the biggest food sources for conventionally reared farm animals. This unnatural diet, paired with their lack of exercise and being on a permanent fat gain diet will change the composition of the animal's fat. This fat is richer, but also lower in healthy Omega 3s and cholesterol, and higher in toxins. If we want to get enough good fats, we must eat fat from animals which have led healthy lives.

We must also give serious thought to our Omega 3 to Omega 6 ratio. For most people, the biggest concern is reducing their intake of Omega 6 and eating more Omega 3. This is because their diets are high in processed fats, both animal and seed-based, which gives them an excess of Omega 6. Having too much

Omega 6 can be oxidizing to the body, and we need Omega 3 to balance it out. But Omega 3 is only found in large quantities in a few rare seeds, fish, and naturally raised animals. So the average person has a poor ratio. But it is possible to have a poor ratio in the opposite direction, especially when you are aiming to eat healthy. If you focus too heavily on animal products and neglect plant fats, you could end up with too much Omega 3 and too little Omega 6, a state that, based on laboratory studies of people taking high doses of Omega 3 supplements, is also oxidizing.

But the problem of not eating enough vegetables goes beyond just Omega ratios. Many people use low carb diets as an excuse to stop eating vegetables all together, which is a big mistake which will cost you your health in the long term. This is where the other two rules for a healthy long-term ketogenic diet become relevant. It is perfectly possible to lose weight in a safe and controlled manner by living off healthy, natural muscle meats and eggs for a week or two. But it is not possible to stay healthy on that diet for a long time, because it is lacking in two things: micronutrients, and dietary fibre.

Micronutrients are the word we use to refer to vitamins, minerals, and antioxidants, which may be vitamins or minerals, but may also be other types of compound. Whereas the macronutrients, fat, carbohydrates, protein, and alcohol, provide building blocks for our bodies and fuel, micronutrients help our cells to stay healthy by reversing cell ageing, reducing oxidation, and protecting cell walls. This can result in health benefits ranging from nice skin to a reduced risk of cancer. For these reasons, we need to eat a wide range of micronutrients every single day. And muscle meat is very low in most micronutrients, especially vitamins and antioxidants. To get vitamins and antioxidants, you have five choices: organ meats, berries, leafy greens, nonsweet fruits, and/or roots.

Organ meats, or offal, are exactly what the name suggests: the organs of animals. Unlike muscle meats, that have a few minerals and little else, organ meats are rich in vitamins and minerals. This is because organs are where micronutrients are used and stored, so when we eat them we are getting a super concentrated dose. There are many organ meats to choose from, and the fewer plants you eat, the more varied your selection of organs must become. Liver, kidneys, tongue, sweetbreads, and bone marrow from many animals are widely available. You also eat organs every time you eat whole fish or shellfish. The two main problems with getting your micronutrients exclusively from offal are its low vitamin C content and high vitamin A content. It can be difficult to maintain this balance without using plants.

Berries are great for us, but on a ketogenic diet you want to minimize the carbs and maximize the micronutrients in them. The berries highest in micronutrients are actually bitter or sour, and have a dusty appearance to their skin. This group includes blueberries, goji berries, black grapes, raspberries, mulberries, and elderberries. These berries have high concentrations of both vitamin C and antioxidants, with a very low carb content. This means that you only need to eat a handful a day to improve your health without leaving ketosis.

Leafy greens like kale, spinach, cabbage, and swiss chard are a wonderful food for their micronutrient content too. Choose dark, bitter, or sour greens above mild ones, as mild ones have fewer antioxidants. If you are not sure about eating berries, either due to their taste or their potential carb content, then leafy greens are a great place to start. One caveat is that you must cook your leafy greens very well to access all the nutrients in them, as these nutrients are encased in cellulose, a plant fibre that our stomach cannot digest. By cooking it we encourage it to release the nutrients we need.

Nonsweet fruits is the term we give to fruits that do not have a high sugar or starch content. Nonsweet fruits include ones like tomatoes, lemons, or squash, but also fatty fruits, like avocados. Remember that fatty fruits may have a high carb content in theory, but most of these carbs are fibre, and that the digestible carbs per 100g are under 5g. Nonsweet fruits carry all the micronutrient benefits of sweet fruit with none of the carb loads, so try and eat a variety of brightly coloured nonsweet fruit every day, preferably raw.

Low carbohydrate root and bulb vegetables, like jicama, onions, garlic, carrots, ginger, turnips, radishes, swede, and celeriac, are packed with amazing nutrients and usually incredibly low in carbs. These parts of the plant are designed to store nutrients, so they are very much like eating offal in that regard. However they are also very good to eat raw, unlike leafy greens, and filling and varied in their uses. These plants also make excellent substitutes for carbohydrate foods like potatoes and pasta.

The last four of these five foods are also very important for their fibre content. Fibre is a sort of carbohydrate which we cannot digest on our own. This means that it will not be turned into glucose in our blood and will not push us out of ketosis. Instead, it feeds the bacteria in our guts. And when our good gut bacteria get fed, we reap the rewards. First of all, a large population of good gut bacteria will cleanse our colon. They encourage peristalsis and make up the bulk of our feces, pushing out invasive bacteria and excess candida yeasts. This will keep our guts fit and healthy.

These gut bacteria also produce waste of their own. When our gut bacteria digest fibre, they produce short chain fatty acids, a type of fat, as you may have guessed from the name. These fats are excellent fuel for our bodies, and happen to be what a lot of larger herbivores, like gorillas, live off. Although we could never live off greens like our cousin the gorilla, we still get plenty of energy from the short chain fatty acids that our gut bacteria release after digesting fibre.

A high fibre intake also regulates the speed of our gut transit. If our gut is moving too fast, the added bulk slows it right down, improving water absorption and encouraging our bodies to absorb as many nutrients and short chain fatty acids as they can. All this leads to better hydration and better health. But if our gut is moving too slow, the fibre adds bulk, moving things along, and irritates the lining of the gut, encouraging lubrication and peristalsis. In short, fibre makes our guts work more efficiently. It is not for nothing that a high fibre intake reduces our chances of bowel cancer.

In summary, therefore, when we are looking at a ketogenic diet for maintaining our weight and health, we must ensure that we eat enough healthy, balanced fats, and plenty of low carb plants, to ensure that we get the right stuff to avoid malnutrition. Although we can in theory live off meat alone, it cannot just be muscle meat, and it will be very hard to balance the right amounts and types of offal to ensure we are getting enough of every micronutrient. Instead, it is far simpler to make sure that we eat berries, nonsweet fruits, leafy greens, root vegetables, and bulb vegetables every day.

Chapter 8: Ketogenic Breakfast Recipes

Squash and Sausage Omelet with Kale

Ingredients:

2 Eggs

1 cup of Kale, chopped

4 oz. Sausage, chopped

2 tbsp Ricotta Cheese

4 ounces Roasted Squash

1 tbsp Olive Oil

Salt and Black Pepper, to taste

Fresh parsley to garnish

Preparation:

1.   Beat the eggs in a bowl, season with salt and pepper and stir in the kale and the ricotta.

2.   In another bowl, mash the squash.

3.   Add the squash to the egg mixture.

4.   Heat ¼ tbsp. of olive oil in a pan over medium heat.

5.   Add sausage and cook until browned on all sides, turning occasionally.

6.   Drizzle the remaining olive oil. Pour the egg mixture over.

7.   Cook for about 2 minutes per side until the eggs are thoroughly cooked and lightly browned.

8.   Remove the pan and run a spatula around the edges of the omelet; slide it onto a warm platter.

9.   Fold in half, and serve sprinkled with fresh parsley.

Sausage Quiche with Tomatoes

Ingredients:

6 Eggs

12 ounces Raw Sausage Roll

10 Cherry Tomatoes, halved

2 tbsp Heavy Cream

2 tbsp Parmesan Cheese

¼ tsp Salt

A pinch of Black Pepper

2 tbsp chopped Parsley

5 Eggplant Slices

Cooking Spray

Preparation:

1.   Preheat your oven to 375 degrees F.

2.   Grease a pie dish (preferably an 8-inch one) with cooking spray.

3.   Press the sausage roll at the bottom of a pie dish.

4.   Arrange the eggplant slices on top of the sausage. Top with cherry tomatoes.

5.   Whisk together the eggs along with the heavy cream, salt, parmesan, and black pepper.

6.   Spoon the egg mixture over the sausage.

7.   Bake for about 40 minutes until it is browned around the edges.

8.   Serve warm and scatter with chopped parsley.

Italian Omelet

Ingredients:

2 Eggs

6 basil Leaves

2 ounces Mozzarella

1 tbsp Butter

1 tbsp Water

5-8 thin slices Chorizo

5 thin slices Tomato (1 tomato)

Salt and Pepper, to taste

Preparation:

1.   Whisk the eggs along with the water and some salt and pepper.

2.   Melt the butter in a skillet and cook the eggs for 30 seconds.

3.   Spread the meat slices over.

4.   Arrange the sliced tomato and mozzarella over the chorizo.

5.   Cook for about 3 minutes. Cover the skillet and continue cooking for 3 more minutes until omelet is completely set.

6.   When ready, remove the pan from heat; run a spatula around the edges of the frittata and flip it onto a warm plate, folded side down.

7.   Serve garnished with basil leaves and green salad.

Ham and Egg Cups

Ingredients:

2 cups chopped Ham

⅓ cup grated Parmesan Cheese

1 tbsp chopped Parsley

¼ cup Almond Flour

9 Eggs

⅓ cup Mayonnaise, sugar-free

¼ tsp Garlic Powder

¼ cup chopped Onion

Sea salt to taste

Cooking Spray

Preparation:

1.   Preheat your oven to 375 degrees F.

2.   Lightly grease nine muffin pans with cooking spray and set aside.

3.   Place the onion, ham, garlic powder, and salt, in a food processor, and pulse until ground. Stir in the mayonnaise, almond flour, and Parmesan cheese.

4.   Press this mixture into the muffin cups.

5.   Make sure it goes all the way up the muffin sides so that there will be room for the egg. Bake for 5 minutes.

6.   Crack an egg into each muffin cup.

7.   Return to the oven and bake for 20 more minutes or until the tops are firm to the touch and eggs are cooked.

8.   Leave to cool slightly before serving and serve right now. Enjoy!

Pesto Mug Muffin Sandwich with Bacon and Cream Cheese

Ingredients:

¼ cup Flax Meal

1 Egg

2 tbsp Heavy Cream

2 tbsp Pesto

¼ cup Almond Flour

¼ tsp Baking Soda

Salt and ground black pepper, to taste

Filling:

2 tbsp Cream Cheese

4 sliced of Bacon

½ medium Avocado, sliced

Preparation:

1. Mix together the dry muffin ingredients in a bowl. Add egg, heavy cream, and pesto, and whisk well with a fork. Season with salt and pepper.

2. Divide the mixture between two ramekins.

3.   Place in the microwave and cook for 60-90 seconds.

4.   Leave to cool slightly before filling.

5.   Meanwhile, in a nonstick skillet, over medium heat, cook the bacon slices until crispy. Transfer to paper towels to soak up excess fat. Set aside.

6.   Invert the muffins onto a plate and cut in half, crosswise.

7.   Assemble the sandwiches by spreading cream cheese and topping with bacon and avocado slices.

Herbed Buttered Eggs

Ingredients:

1 tbsp Coconut Oil

2 tbsp Butter

1 tsp fresh Thyme

4 Eggs

2 Garlic Cloves, minced

½ cup chopped Parsley

½ cup chopped Cilantro

¼ tsp Cumin

¼ tsp Cayenne Pepper

Salt and ground black pepper, to taste

Preparation:

1.　　　Drizzle the coconut oil into a non-stick skillet over medium heat.

2.　　　Once the oil is warm, add the butter, leave to melt.

3.　　　Add garlic and thyme and cook for 30 seconds.

4.　　　Sprinkle with parsley and cilantro, and cook for another 2-3 minutes, until crisp.

5.　　　Carefully crack the eggs into the skillet.

6.　　　Lower the heat and cook for 4-6 minutes. Adjust the seasoning.

7.　　　When the eggs are just set, turn the heat off and transfer to a serving plate.

8.　　　Serve warm.

Breakfast Hash with Bacon and Zucchini

Ingredients:

1 Medium Zucchini, diced

2 Bacon Slices

1 Egg

1 tbsp Coconut Oil

½ small Onion, chopped

1 tbsp chopped Parsley

¼ tsp Salt

Preparation:

1.   Place the bacon in a skillet and cook over medium heat for a few minutes, until the bacon is crispy. Remove from the skillet and set aside.

2.   Warm the coconut oil and cook the onion until soft, for about 3-4 minutes, stirring occasionally.

3.   Add the zucchini, and cook for 10 more minutes until zucchini is brown and tender, but not mushy. Transfer to a plate and season with salt.

4.   Crack the egg into the same skillet and fry it over medium heat.

5.   Top the zucchini mixture with the bacon slices and a fried egg.

6.   Serve hot, sprinkled with parsley.

Omelet Wrap with Avocado and Salmon

Ingredients:

½ Avocado, sliced

2 tbsp chopped Chives

½ package smoked Salmon (about 1.8 ounces), cut into strips

1 Spring Onion, sliced

3 Eggs

2 tbsp Cream Cheese

1 tbsp Butter

Salt and pepper, to taste

Preparation:

1.	In a small bowl, combine the chives and cream cheese. Set aside.

2.	Now, beat the eggs in a large bowl and season with salt and pepper.

3.	Melt the butter in a pan over medium heat.

4.	Add the eggs to the pan and cook for about 3 minutes.

5.	Carefully flip the omelet over and continue cooking for another 2 minutes until golden.

6.	Remove the omelet to a plate and spread the chive mixture over.

7.	Arrange the salmon, avocado, and onion slices. Wrap the omelet.

8.	Serve immediately.

Feta and Spinach Frittata with Cherry Tomatoes

Ingredients:

5 ounces Spinach

8 ounces crumbled Feta Cheese

1 pint halved Cherry Tomatoes

10 Eggs

3 tbsp Olive Oil

4 Scallions, diced

Salt and pepper, to taste

Preparation:

1.   Preheat your oven to 350 degrees F.

2.   Drizzle the oil in a 2-quart casserole and place in the oven until heated.

3.   In a bowl, whisk the eggs along with the pepper and salt until thoroughly combined.

4.   Stir in the spinach, feta cheese, and scallions.

5.   Pour the mixture into the casserole, top with the cherry tomatoes and place back in the oven. Bake for 25 minutes until your frittata is set in the middle.

6.   When done, remove the casserole from the oven and run a spatula around the edges of the frittata; slide it onto a warm platter.

7.   Cut the frittata into wedges and serve with salad.

Almond Butter Shake

Ingredients:

1 ½ cup Almond Milk

2 tbsp Almond Butter

⅛ tsp Almond Extract

½ tsp Cinnamon

2 tbsp Flax Meal

1 scoop Collagen Peptides

A pinch of Salt

15 drops of Stevia

A handful of Ice Cubes

Preparation:

1.   Add almond milk, almond butter, flax meal, almond extract, collagen peptides, a pinch of salt, and stevia to the bowl of your blender.

2.   Blitz until uniform and smooth, for about 30 seconds.

3.   Add a bit more almond milk if it's very thick.

4.   Then taste, and adjust flavor as needed, adding more stevia for sweetness or almond butter to creaminess.

5.   Pour into your smoothie glass, add the ice cubes and sprinkle with cinnamon.

6.   Enjoy!

Quick Breakfast Porridge

Ingredients:

½ tsp Vanilla Extract

½ cup Water

1 tbsp Chia Seeds

2 tbsp Hemp Seeds

1 tbsp Flaxseed Meal

2 tbsp Almond Meal

2 tbsp Shredded Coconut

¼ tsp Granulated Stevia

1 tbsp Walnuts, chopped

Preparation:

1.   Put the chia seeds, hemp seeds, flaxseed meal, almond meal, granulated stevia, and shredded coconut in a nonstick saucepan and pour over the water.

2.   Simmer over medium heat, stirring occasionally, until creamed and thickened, for about 3-4 minutes. Stir in vanilla.

3.   When the porridge is ready, spoon into a serving bowl, sprinkle with chopped walnuts and serve warm.

Mint Chocolate Protein Shake

Ingredients:

3 cups Flax Milk, chilled

3 tsp unsweetened Cocoa Powder

1 medium Avocado, pitted, peeled, and sliced

1 cup Coconut Milk, chilled

3 Mint Leaves + extra to garnish

3 tbsp Erythritol or more as desired

1 scoop low carb Protein Powder

Whipping cream for topping

Directions:

1.   Combine the milk, cocoa powder, avocado, coconut milk, mint leaves, erythritol, and protein powder into the smoothie maker, and blend for 1 minute to smooth.

2.   Pour the drink into serving cups, lightly add some whipping cream on top of them, and garnish with 1 or 2 mint leaves.

3.   Serve immediately.

Simple Egg Cups

Ingredients:

4 eggs

1/2 cup cheddar cheese, shredded

1 cup mix vegetables, diced

1/2 cup mozzarella cheese, shredded

2 tbsp cilantro, chopped

1/4 cup half and half

Pepper

Salt

Directions:

1.   Add all ingredients except mozzarella cheese into the mixing bowl and mix well.

2.   Pour egg mixture into the four halfpint wide mouth jars. Place lids on top but do not seal.

3.   Pour 2 cups water into the instant pot then place trivet into the pot.

4.   Place egg jars on a trivet.

5.   Seal pot with lid and cook on high pressure for 5 minutes.

6.   Release pressure using quick release method than open the lid carefully.

7.   Carefully remove egg jars from instant pot and top with shredded mozzarella cheese and broil until cheese melted.

8.   Serve and enjoy.

Bacon Frittata

Ingredients:

6 eggs

1/2 tsp Italian seasoning

2 1/2 tbsp heavy cream

1/4 cup bacon, cooked and chopped

1/2 cup tomato, chopped

1 cup fresh spinach

1/4 tsp pepper

1/4 tsp salt

Directions:

1.   In a bowl, whisk eggs with spices and heavy cream.

2.   Spray 7" baking pan with cooking spray.

3.   Add bacon, tomato, and spinach to the pan. Pour egg mixture over the bacon mixture.

4.   Cover pan with aluminum foil piece.

5.   Pour 1 ½ cups of water into the instant pot then place trivet to the pot.

6.   Place baking pan on top of the trivet. Seal instant pot with lid and cook on manual high pressure for 15 minutes.

7.   Release pressure using quick release method than open the lid.

8.   Serve and enjoy.

Almond Pancake

Ingredients:

1 egg

1 1/2 tbsp olive oil

3/4 tsp baking powder

3 tbsp swerve

1 cup almond flour

1 1/4 cups coconut milk

3/4 tsp baking soda

Directions:

1.   In a large mixing bowl, mix together flour, baking soda, baking powder, and swerve.

2.   Add buttermilk, oil, and eggs and whisk until well combined.

3.   Spray 7" springform pan with cooking spray. Pour batter into the prepared pan.

4.   Pour 1 cup water into the instant pot then place a trivet in the pot.

5.   Place pan on top of the trivet.

6.   Seal pot with lid and cook on low pressure for 17 minutes.

7   Release pressure using quick release method than open the lid carefully.

8.   Remove pan from the pot and set aside to cool completely.

9.   Slice and serve.

Bacon Brussels sprouts

Ingredients:

1 lb Brussels sprouts, trimmed and halved

1/2 cup orange juice

2 bacon slices, diced

1 tbsp olive oil

2 tsp orange zest

1/2 cup water

Directions:

1.   Add olive oil to the instant pot and set the pot on sauté mode.

2.   Add bacon and sauté for 35 minutes or until crisp.

3.   Add water and orange juice and deglaze the instant pot.

4.   Add Brussels sprouts and stir well.

5.   Seal pot with lid and cook on manual high pressure for 3 minutes.

6.   Release pressure using quick release method than open the lid.

7.   Top with orange zest and serve.

Breakfast Quiche

Ingredients:

8 eggs

1 1/2 cup mozzarella cheese, shredded

1/2 cup almond flour

1/2 cup almond milk

1/4 tsp pepper

2 green onions, chopped

1 cup tomatoes, chopped

1 red pepper, chopped

1/4 tsp salt

Directions:

1.   Place trivet into the bottom of the instant pot.

2.   Pour 1 cup water into the instant pot.

3.   In a large bowl, whisk eggs, flour, milk, pepper, and salt.

4.   Add vegetables and cheese and stir until combined.

5.   Pour egg mixture into the dish that will fit inside your instant pot.

6.   Cover dish with foil and place on the trivet.

7.   Seal instant pot with lid and select manual high pressure for 30 minutes.

8.   Allow to release pressure naturally for 10 minutes then release using quick release method.

9.   Carefully remove the dish from the instant pot.

10.   Serve and enjoy.

Mushroom Cheese Chive Omelet

Ingredients:

5 eggs, lightly beaten

1/2 tbsp cheddar cheese

2 tbsp butter

1 onion, chopped

2 tbsp chives, minced

1 bell pepper, chopped

1 1/2 cups mushrooms, sliced

1/2 cup coconut milk

Directions:

1.   Add butter into the instant pot and set the pot on sauté mode.

2.   In a bowl, whisk eggs until well combined.

3.   Add remaining ingredients and mix well. Pour egg mixture into the instant pot and cook for 2 minutes.

4.   Seal pot with lid and select manual high pressure for 8 minutes.

5.   Release pressure using quick release method than open the lid.

6.   Serve and enjoy.

Kale Egg Cheese Breakfast

Ingredients:

3 eggs

1 tsp herb de Provence

1/2 cup cheddar cheese, shredded

1/2 cup kale, chopped

1/4 cup heavy cream

1/2 cup bacon slices, chopped

1/2 small onion, chopped

Pepper

Salt

Directions:

1.   In a large bowl, whisk together egg and heavy cream.

2.   Add kale, bacon, cheddar cheese, herb de Provence, pepper, and salt. Stir well.

3.   Pour egg mixture into the baking dish.

4.   Pour 1 cup of water into the instant pot and place trivet in the pot.

5.   Place baking dish on top of the trivet.

6.   Seal pot with lid and cook on high for 20 minutes.

7.   Allow to release pressure naturally then open the lid.

8.   Serve and enjoy.

Delicious Carrot Muffins

Ingredients:

3 eggs

1 1/2 cups water

1/2 cup heavy cream

1 tsp apple pie spice

1 cup shredded carrot

1/3 cup Truvia

1 tsp baking powder

1/4 cup coconut oil, melted

1 cup almond flour

1/2 cup pecans, chopped

Directions:

1.   Pour water into the instant pot then place a trivet in the pot.

2.   Add all ingredients except pecans and carrots into the large bowl and using electric mixer blend until fluffy.

3.   Add carrots and pecans and fold well.

4.   Pour batter into the silicone muffin cups and place on top of the trivet.

5.   Seal pot with lid and cook on high for 20 minutes.

6.   Release pressure using quick release method than open the lid.

7.   Serve and enjoy.

Healthy Pumpkin Bread

Ingredients:

2 eggs, lightly beaten

1 tbsp almond butter, melted

1/4 cup almond milk

1 cup almond flour

1/2 cup pumpkin puree

1/4 tsp turmeric powder

1/2 tsp pumpkin pie spice

1/4 tsp nutmeg

1/2 tsp salt

Directions:

1.   In a large bowl, combine together almond flour, pumpkin pie spice, turmeric, nutmeg, baking powder, and salt.

2.   Add pumpkin puree, eggs, and almond milk into the almond flour mixture and stir until well combined.

3.   Spray springform pan with cooking spray.

4.   Pour bread batter into the prepared pan and cover with foil.

5.   Pour 1 cup of water into the instant pot then place a trivet in the pot.

6.   Place pan on top of the trivet.

7.   Seal pot with lid and cook on low for 25 minutes.

8.   Allow to release pressure naturally then open the lid.

9   Cut bread into the slices and serve.

Chapter 9: Ketogenic Lunch Recipes

Garlicky Chicken Livers

Ingredients:

½ lb. chicken liver

1 tsp. lemon juice

2 tbsps. olive oil

2 tbsps. melted ghee

3 cloves garlic

Salt

Directions:

1.   Wash the chicken livers. Trim and dry them.

2.   Dry-fry them in a nonstick frying pan for about 4 minutes without the use of oil.

3.   To the pan, add lemon juice, ghee-olive oil, and salt to taste. Stir once to mix.

4.   Sprinkle the garlic and serve.

Chicken Bacon Wraps

Ingredients:

12 skinless and boneless chicken breast halves

12 slices of bacon

16 oz. chive and onion cream cheese

12 tbsps. divided olive oil spread

Salt

Directions:

1. Flatten the chicken breasts to 1/2-inch thickness.

2. Spread 3 tablespoons of cream cheese over each chicken breast.

3. Dot with 1 tablespoon olive oil spread and sprinkle with the salt; roll up and wrap each rolled piece with a bacon strip.

4. Grease your pan and place chicken onto it and bake uncovered for about 40 minutes at 400 degrees F or until the juices run clear.

5. Transfer the pan 6 inches from the heat source; broil for 5 minutes until the bacon is crispy.

Cauliflower Salad

Ingredients:

Salad:

   1 head cauliflower, medium

   1½ c. mushrooms, sliced

   1½ tbsps. olive oil

   1 tsp. fresh dill

   1 tsp. chives, chopped

   ½ tsp. paprika, smoked

   Salt

   Pepper

Sauce:

   ½ c. extra-virgin olive oil

   ¼ c. soy milk, unsweetened

   1 tsp. cider vinegar, raw

   Salt

   White pepper

Directions:

1. Make the salad; cut cauliflower into tiny florets.
2. Place the cauliflower florets into a pan and cover with water.
3. Bring to a boil and reduce heat. Simmer for 3-4 minutes or until crisp-tender.
4. In the meantime, heat olive oil in a skillet. Cook mushrooms for 5-8 minutes or until soft. Toss in the cauliflower and shake to coat with oil. Season to taste with salt and pepper.
5. Make the sauce; make sure oil and milk are equal temperatures. It is a significant step.
6. Place soy milk, cider vinegar, and seasonings in a food blender. Blend until smooth. While the blender is running low, gradually stream in extra-virgin olive oil.
7. Blend until thickens.
8. In a bowl, toss cauliflower with prepared sauce, dill, and chives.
9. Divide between bowls and sprinkle with paprika. Chill briefly before serving.

Salt-and-Pepper Stir-Fried Shrimp

Ingredients:

- 4 cloves garlic, chopped

- 2 tsps. divided salt

- 2 tbsps. vegetable

- 2 lbs. shrimp

- ½ tsp. Red peppercorn

- ½ tsp. white peppercorn

- ½ tsp. black peppercorn

- ½ tsp. green peppercorn

- 1 c. chopped cilantro leaves

Directions:

1.   Crush the peppercorns in a mortar.

2.   Into a large bowl, place the shrimp, salt and half of the crushed peppercorns; toss to coat the shrimp evenly and set aside.

3.   Heat a large nonstick pan over high heat. Add the garlic, oil, and the remaining peppercorns and salt; cook for about 1 minute, continually stirring, until fragrant.

4.   Add the shrimp to the mixture and cook for about 4 minutes as you stir.

5.   Add the cilantro; turn off the heat; and toss to combine.

6.   Serve right away.

Almond Buns

Ingredients:

   2 eggs

   ¾ c. almond flour

   5 tbsps. Butter, unsalted

   1½ tsp. baking powder

   1½ tsp. stevia or Splenda

Directions:

1.   Combine the dry ingredients in a bowl.

2.   Whisk in the eggs.

3.   Melt butter and add it to the mixture.

4.   Divide the mixture into equal 6 parts; place into a muffin top pan or something similar

5.   Bake at 350 degrees F for about 12-17 minutes. You may need to watch the first time you make these since cooking time will vary depending on your oven.

6.   Let cool on a wire rack.

Stuffed Portabella with Nut Pate

Ingredients:

4 portabella mushrooms caps

1 tbsp. olive oil

1 tbsp. coconut aminos

Pepper

Salt

Nut pate:

1 c. soaked macadamia nuts

1 tbsp. coconut aminos

1 chopped celery stalk

Kosher salt

Directions:

1.   Heat oven to 375F and line a baking sheet with parchment paper.

2.   In a bowl, beat olive oil with coconut aminos. Brush in mushroom caps with oil mixture and arrange onto a baking sheet.

3.   Bake for 15 minutes.

4.   In the meantime, make the nut paste; rinse and drain macadamia nuts. Place the macadamia nuts and celery in a food processor and process until just smooth. In the last seconds of processing, add coconut aminos and salt to taste.

5.   Process until the coconut aminos is incorporated.

6.   Remove the portabella from the oven and place on a plate. Fill with macadamia pate and serve warm.

Creamy Cauliflower Soup

Ingredients:

2 c. cauliflower florets

2 c. wild mushrooms, sliced

2 c. coconut milk, full-fat

2 tbsps. avocado oil

1 tsp. celery flakes, dried

½ tbsps. Thyme, freshly chopped

1 minced clove garlic

Salt

Pepper

Directions:

1.   In a saucepan, mix celery flakes, cauliflower, and coconut milk.

2.   Cover and bring to a boil over medium-high heat.

3.   Reduce heat and simmer for 6-7 minutes. Kill the heat and puree using an immersion blender.

4.   In the meantime, heat avocado oil in a skillet. Add thyme and garlic. Cook until fragrant. Toss in wild mushrooms and cook for 6-7 minutes or until tender.

5.   Pour in pureed cauliflower and bring to a boil. Reduce heat and simmer 6-8 minutes or until thickened.

6.   Serve warm with Keto bread.

Spicy Garlic Butter Shrimp

Ingredients:

4 lbs. large-sized shrimp, unpeeled

2 tbsps. garlic, minced

½ c. butter

Lemon pepper seasoning

Garlic powder

Directions:

1.   Preheat the oven to 300 degrees F.

2.   Mix the butter and the garlic.

3.   Place the shrimp in a saucepan and dot with the garlic butter; sprinkle well with the garlic powder and the lemon pepper.

4.   In an open state, bake for about 30 minutes, stirring once or twice, until the shrimp are opaque, making sure the shrimp is evenly cooked.

5.   Serve alongside the butter sauce that is in a separate bowl or the one containing the shrimp for dipping.

6.   You may serve alongside cauliflower rice.

Sticky Drumsticks

Ingredients:

- 8 chicken drumsticks

- ½ c. olive oil

- ¼ c. sweet chili sauce

- 2 garlic cloves, minced

- ¼ c. soy sauce

- 2 tsps. sesame seeds

Directions:

1. Slice through the thickest part of each drumstick using a sharp knife. Arrange them in a glass dish.

2. In a bowl, mix the sauces and garlic. Rub all over the drumstick; marinate for about 30 minutes in the refrigerator.

3. Preheat the oven to 248 degrees F of 356 for the fan.

4. Place the drumsticks on a nonstick baking paper. Sprinkle them with sesame seeds. Bake for about 45 minutes. Let cool slightly; serve.

Grilled Spicy Lime Shrimp

Ingredients:

- 1 lb. peeled and deveined medium shrimp

- 1 juiced lime

- ½ c. vegetable oil

- 3 tbsps. Cajun seasoning

Directions:

1. In a Ziploc bag, mix the Cajun seasoning, lime juice, and vegetable oil. Add the shrimp, shake to coat, squeeze out the excess air, seal the bag, and marinate for 20 minutes in the refrigerator.

2. Preheat an outdoor grill to medium heat. Lightly grease the grate.

3. Take the shrimp from marinade as you shake off any excess; discard marinade.

4. Allow cooking both sides for 2 minutes each. Serve.

Instant Pot Olive Steamed Fish

Ingredients:

- 4 white fish fillets
- 1 c. pitted and chopped olives
- 1 lb. halved cherry tomatoes
- ½ tsp. dried thyme
- 1 minced garlic clove
- Olive oil
- Salt
- Black pepper
- 1 c. water

Directions:

1.   Put the water in your instant pot.

2.   Put fish fillets in the steamer basket of the pot.

3.   Add tomatoes and olives on top.

4.   Also add garlic, thyme, oil, salt, and pepper.

5.   Cook on Low for 10 minutes while the pot is covered.

6.   Release the pressure, uncover the pot, divide fish, olives and tomatoes mix among plates and serve. Enjoy!

Coconut Milk Beef Curry

Ingredients:

- 2 lbs. cubed beef steak
- 2 tbsps. Extra virgin olive oil
- 3 diced potatoes
- 1 tbsp. wine mustard
- 2½ tbsps. Curry powder
- 2 chopped yellow onions
- 2 minced garlic cloves
- 10 oz. canned coconut milk
- 2 tbsps. Tomato sauce
- Salt

- Black pepper

Directions:

1.   Set your instant pot on Sauté mode, add the oil and heat it up.

2.   Add onions and garlic, stir and cook for 4 minutes.

3.   Add potatoes and mustard, stir and cook for 1 minute.

4.   Add beef, stir and brown on all sides. Add curry powder, salt, and pepper, stir and cook for 2 minutes.

5.   Add coconut milk and tomato sauce, stir, cover the pot and cook at High for 10 minutes. Release the pressure, uncover the pot, divide curry among plates and serve.

Ginger Short Ribs

Ingredients:

2 chopped green onions

1 tsp. vegetable oil

3 minced garlic cloves

3 slices of ginger

4 lbs. short ribs

½ c. water

½ c. soy sauce

¼ c. rice wine

¼ c. pear juice

2 tsps. Sesame oil

Directions:

1.   Set your instant pot on Sauté mode, add the oil and heat it up.

2.   Add green onions, ginger and garlic, stir and cook for 1 minute.

3.   Add ribs, water, wine, soy sauce, sesame oil and pear juice, stir and cook for 2-3 minutes.

4.   Cover the pot and cook at High for 45 minutes.

5.   Release the pressure naturally for 15 minutes, uncover the pot and transfer the ribs to a plate.

6.   Strain liquid from the pot, divide ribs among plates and drizzle the sauce all over.

Steak and Salsa

Ingredients:

- 1 diced beef tomatoes
- 1 tbsp. olive oil
- ½ diced red onion
- ½ bunch chopped cilantro
- Salt
- Pepper
- 1 lb. sliced stewing beef
- 1 sliced bell pepper
- ½ sliced onion
- 4 tbsps. Butter
- 2 tbsps. Mixed dry seasoning:
- 1 tsp. cumin
- ½ tsp. sweet paprika
- ½ tsp. paprika flakes
- 1 tsp. garlic salt
- ½ tsp. black pepper

Directions:

1.   Cover bottom of crock-pot with the salsa.

2.   Add remaining ingredients and mix well.

3.   Cover, cook on low for 6-8 hours.

Chili Beef Stew

Ingredients:

   3 lbs. stewing beef

   2 cans Italian tomatoes

   1 c. beef broth

   4 tbsps. Butter

   1 tsp. Cayenne pepper

   1 tbsp. Worcestershire sauce

   1 tsp. oregano, dried

   1 tsp. thyme, dried

   Salt

   Pepper

Directions:

1.   Add all the ingredients to the crock-pot, mix well.

2.   Cover, cook on high for 6 hours.

3.   Break up the beef with a fork, pull apart in the crock-pot.

4.   Taste and adjust the seasoning, if needed.

5.   Re-cover, cook for an additional 2 hours on low.

Chapter 10: Ketogenic Dinner Recipes

Chicken Cacciatore with Spaghetti Squash

Ingredients:

4 skinless chicken thighs

1 medium diced Onion

1 bell peppers

2 minced cloves Garlic

½ tsp. thyme, dried

1 c. Chicken stock

28 oz. tomatoes, diced

8 oz. Tomato sauce

½ tsp. dried basil

Salt

Pepper

½ diced yellow squash

½ tsp. dried oregano

1 Spaghetti squash

Directions:

1. Dice the veggies. Set them aside.
2. Cut the chicken up. Season it as desired.
3. Place the chicken in a Dutch oven and let it brown for about 8 minutes.
4. Add in the onion, garlic and bell pepper and let them cook for approximately 5 minutes or until the onions soften.
5. Add the chicken tomato sauce, tomatoes, and the chicken stock.
6. Season as desired and mix well before letting everything boil.
7. Turn the heat to low and let everything cook for 30 minutes.
8. Add the yellow squash. Cook between 15 and 30 more minutes.

Meat-Based Pizza

Ingredients:

Small package of Ground uncooked beef

Salsa

1 diced Onion

Italian Spices

Garlic powder

Shredded Mozzarella cheese

6 strips Bacon

Directions:

1.   Dice onion and put the onion into a baking dish.

2.   Add the beef, salsa, garlic powder and other spices into a baking dish. Mix together.

3.   Shred the cheese and put it evenly over the top of the beef mixture.

4.   Cut the bacon into small pieces and put the pieces on top of the cheese.

5.   Ensure your oven is set to 375 degrees F

6.   Place the pizza in the oven and let it cook for 35 minutes.

Mexican Casserole

Ingredients:

½ tsp. Cumin

1 head Cauliflower

½ white Onion

½ tsp. Chili powder

1 Green bell pepper

1½ c. Parmesan

1 hashed Bell pepper

4 chopped Cherry tomatoes

Directions:

1.   Ensure your oven is set to 350 degrees Fahrenheit.

2.   Place the skillet on top of the stove over a burner set to medium heat.

3.   Roast the chili powder, pepper, cumin, and onion, stirring regularly until the veggies are fully cooked.

4.   Dice the cauliflower.   Cook it in the microwave for 3 minutes.

5.   Put the tomatoes and 1 cup of the cheese in with the cauliflower. Mix.

6.   Mix the results with the vegetables.

7.   Using cooking spray coat a baking dish.

8.   Add the vegetable mixture to the baking dish.

9.   Add the rest of the cheese.

10.   Place the dish in the oven and let it cook for approximately 40 minutes.

11.   Garnish as desired.

Tasty Fried Chicken Breast

Ingredients:

    1 Chicken breast

    Butter

    Salt

    Pepper

    Curry powder

    Garlic powder

    ½ c. Greens

Directions:

1.   Cut chicken into small chunks.

2.   Heat up the butter in a frying pan.

3.   Put the chicken into the pan. Stir to coat chicken.

4.   Add spices to taste.

5.   Stir-fry until the chicken browns and gets crunchy.

6.   Serve with greens on the side.

Baby-Back Ribs

Ingredients:

   4 lbs. baby back pork ribs

   2 tbsps. sugar

   2 tbsps. chili powder

   ½ tsp. mustard powder

   ½ tsp. thyme leaves, dried

   Salt

Directions:

1.   Preheat the oven to 300F or light an outdoor grill.

2.   In a small bowl, except for the ribs, combine the rest of the ingredients; rub the mixture on each side of the ribs.

3.   If using a grill, cook the ribs with the bone-side down over medium-low heat or when the coals

are covered with ash. Adjust the flame and add coals if necessary; cook for about 1½ hours.

4.   If using an oven, place the ribs with the bone-side down; cook for 1½ hours.

5.   The ribs are cooked when the ribs separate when you insert a fork between them.

Almond-Crusted Tilapia

Ingredients:

   4 (each 6 oz.) tilapia fillets

   2 tbsps. olive oil

   2 tbsps. butter

   ¼ c. tapioca flour

   Salt

   1 c. sliced almonds, divided

Directions:

1.   Place ½ cup of the almonds in the food processor until chopped into beautiful pieces. Transfer into a shallow bowl. Add the flour, mix until combined.

2.   Evenly sprinkle the fillets with salt and dredge with the almond-flour mixture.

3.   In a large skillet, melt the butter with the olive oil over medium heat. Add the fish; cook for about 4 minutes per side or until golden brown. Transfer the fillets into a serving plate.

4.   Add the remaining almond into the skillet; cook for 1 minute, frequently stirring, or until golden.

5.   With a slotted spoon, remove the almonds; sprinkle over the fillets.

Perfect Boneless Pork Tenderloin

Ingredients:

   1 lb. pork tenderloin, boneless

   Onion powder

   Any of the following or a mixture (rosemary, thyme, garlic powder, or savory)

   Salt

   Pepper

Directions:

1.   Determine the exact weight of your roast from the meat wrapper. This will determine how long you need to cook it.

2.   Preheat the oven to 500F.

3.   Season the meat according to your preference. Place uncovered on a shelf in the bottom 1/3 of the oven.

4.   Bake EXACTLY for 5½ minutes PER POUND. Adjust the time according to your oven's heat retention and accuracy.

5.   Turn the oven off. Do not open the door for about 45 minutes to 1 hour. If your oven has a probe thermometer, you can open the oven door when it alerts that the temperature is 140F.

6.   Remove the pork from the oven; cover lightly with foil; and let rest for about 5 -10 minutes to redistribute the internal juices.

Basil Tomato Salmon

Ingredients:

2 boneless salmon fillets

4 tbsps. olive oil

1 thinly sliced tomato

1 tbsp. basil, dried

2 tbsps. Parmesan cheese, grated

Directions:

1.   Preheat the oven to 375F.

2.   Take an aluminum foil and line the baking sheet and grease it with nonstick cooking spray.

3.   Place the salmon on the foil; sprinkle with the basil; top with the tomato; drizzle with the olive oil, or sprinkle with parmesan.

4.   Bake for about 20 minutes, or until the salmon center is opaque and the cheese is lightly browned on top.

Cheesy Tuna Casserole

Ingredients:

12 oz. drained Tuna

16 oz. frozen Green beans

3 oz. sliced fresh mushrooms

2 tbsps. Butter

½ c. Chicken broth

¾ c. Heavy cream

2 chopped Onions

Salt

Pepper

Xanthan gum

1 stalk hashed Celery

8 oz. shredded Cheddar cheese

Directions:

1. Cook the green beans in a medium pot. Drain well.
2. Place the butter, celery, mushrooms, and onion in a pan and place the pan on top of the stove over a burner turned to medium heat and let everything cook for 5 minutes.
3. Add the broth. Boil, letting the liquid cook down by half.
4. Stir in the cream. Let come back up to a boil.
5. Turn down the heat until the sauce is thickened, stirring frequently. Don't let it boil over.
6. Season to taste.
7. Put the mushroom and tuna mixture into the green beans.

8. Add salt and pepper if needed.
9. Put the cheese in it, thoroughly mixing it in.
10. Put the mixture into a 1.5 or 2-quart casserole dish.
11. Microwave or bake until hot.

Ground Beef and Bell Peppers

Ingredients:

1 diced Onion

Coconut oil

1 lb. beef, ground

1 c. freshly chopped Spinach

Salt

Pepper

1 sliced red Bell pepper

Directions:

1. Chop the spinach. Set aside.

2. Dice the onion into tiny pieces.

3. Add the oil to a skillet before placing the skillet on the stove over a burner set to medium heat.

Add in the onion and coat well in oil. Let it cook for 60 seconds.

4.   Mix in the spinach and the beef and stir well. Season as desired.

5.   Stir-fry everything until cooked.

6.   Put the sliced fresh bell pepper on a serving plate, and dish up the cooked meat mixture beside the peppers.

Meat Bacon Tacos

Ingredients:

   1 lb. cooked hamburger

   ½ c. taco sauce

   ¼ c. ranch dressing

   2 c. shredded lettuce, thinly sliced

   ½ c. tomatoes, diced

   20 strips bacon

   2 whisked eggs

Directions:

1.   On a plastic microwave bacon dish, lay out 5 strips of bacon over the cooking mold to form a "taco shell." Brush with egg wash and microwave until it forms a shell, about 4 minutes.

2.   Cook hamburger meat and add ¼ cup taco sauce.

3.   Now add all the ingredients to build a taco. This includes dividing all ingredients into the 4 tacos you will make.

4.   If you do not want all the bacon, you can substitute small torts.

5.   Another possibility is to create a taco bowl out of this by adding the lettuce and diced bacon with all the rest of the ingredients in a small bowl.

6.   Finally, add a dash of tobacco sauce for a bite.

Zucchini & Almond Pesto

Ingredients:

2 cubed medium Zucchinis

1 cubed avocado

¼ c. walnuts

¼ c. basil leaves, fresh

¼ c. almond slices

2 peeled cloves garlic

½ juiced lemon

¼ c. Parmesan cheese, grated

1 tbsp. olive oil

½ tbsp. Italian seasoning

Salt

Pepper

Directions:

1.   This recipe is easy to make. In your food processor, place all the above ingredients and grind until a smooth paste, about 30-45 seconds.

2.   The pesto can be eaten cold like a dip.

3.   You can add the pesto to other recipes for flavor and food enhancement. For example baked chicken with the pesto on top.

Salmon and Veggies

Ingredients:

4 boneless salmon fillets

2 c. water

3 tbsps. Olive oil

1 sliced lemon

1 chopped white onion

3 sliced tomatoes

4 chopped thyme sprigs

4 chopped parsley sprigs

Salt

Black pepper

Directions:

1.   Drizzle the oil on a parchment paper.

2.   Add a layer of tomatoes, salt, and pepper.

3.   Drizzle some oil again, add fish and season with salt and pepper.

4.   Drizzle some more oil, add thyme and parsley, onions, lemon slices, salt and pepper and wrap packet.

5.   Add water to the instant pot, add the steamer basket, add packet inside, cover and cook on High for 15 minutes.

6.   Unwrap packet, divide fish and veggies between plates and serve.

7.   Enjoy!

Shrimp and Turnips

Ingredients:

   2 lbs. deveined shrimp

   1 lb. chopped tomatoes

   1 c. water

   3 quartered turnips

   4 tbsps. olive oil

   4 chopped onions

   1 tsp. ground coriander

   1 tsp. curry powder

   Juice of 1 lemon

   Salt

   Black pepper

Directions:

1.   Put the water in your instant pot, add steamer basket, add turnips, cover pot, cook on High for 6 minutes, drain, transfer to a bowl and leave aside for now.

2.   Clean your instant pot, set it on sauté mode, add oil, heat it up, add onions, stir and cook for 5 minutes.

3.   Add salt, coriander, curry, tomatoes, lemon juice, shrimp, and turnips, stir, cover and cook on High for 6 minutes more.

4.   Divide shrimp into bowls and serve.

5.   Enjoy!

Spaghetti & Meat Squash

Ingredients:

   2 Spaghetti squash

   2 tbsps. coconut oil

   1 lb. ground beef, grass fed

   1 c. Parmesan cheese

   1 tsp. chili powder

   1 tsp. Italian seasoning

½ tsp. oregano

2 minced cloves garlic

3 c. spaghetti sauce

¼ c. coconut flour

Directions:

1.   Set your oven to 350 degrees F and cook spaghetti squash for an hour. Cut the squash into long strips. Add to mixing bowl with coconut flour and coconut oil and gently fold with a spatula until thoroughly mixed.

2.   Next, cook beef with all the spices until brown. Do NOT drain fat and add spaghetti sauce.

3.   Finally place spaghetti squash on the plate first, add parmesan cheese (divide among servings).

4.   Now add spaghetti sauce with meat on top and serve immediately.

5.   You can add pepper flakes or chili spice for more zest.

Lebanese Chicken Thighs

Ingredients:

4 chicken thighs

2 c. water

1 chicken bouillon cube

¼ c. garlic olive oil

2 tbsps. Butter

1 quartered white onion

2 diced carrots

2 diced celery stalks

2 small quartered tomatoes

1 juice of a lemon

¼ c. soy sauce

3 c. diced lettuce and field greens

Directions:

1.   Set oven to high. Mix all ingredients using a mixing bowl and pour over chicken.

2.   Cook for 30 minutes while the bowl is covered.

3.   On a plate put 2 thighs on about 2 cups of the greens and scoop a cup of the broth from the chicken and pour over it.

4.   One variant is to add parmesan cheese over the greens.

5.   Another variant is to add ½ a cup of olives.

6.   Serve immediately.

Chapter 11: Ketogenic Side Dish

Stewed Celery Mix

Ingredients:

1.   1 celery bunch, roughly chopped

2.   1 yellow onion, chopped

3.   1 bunch green onion, chopped

4.   4 garlic cloves, minced

5.   Salt and black pepper to the taste

6.   1 parsley bunch, chopped

7.   2 mint bunches, chopped

8.   2 cups veggie stock

9.   4 tablespoons olive oil

Directions:

1.   Grease your Crockpot with the oil, add celery, onion, green onion, garlic, salt, pepper and stock, cover and cook on Low for 3 hours and 30 minutes. Add parsley and mint, cover and cook on Low for 30

minutes more. Divide between plates and serve as a side dish.

2. Enjoy!

Lemony Collard Greens

Ingredients:

2 garlic cloves, minced

½ cup veggie stock

2 and ½ pounds collard greens, chopped

1 teaspoon lemon juice

1 tablespoon olive oil

Salt and black pepper to the taste

Directions:

1. Grease your Crockpot with the oil, add greens, garlic, stock, lemon juice, salt and pepper, cover and cook on Low for 3 hours. Divide between plates and serve as a side dish.

2.   Enjoy!

Collard Greens, Bacon and Tomatoes

Ingredients:

1 pound collard greens

3 bacon strips, chopped

¼ cup cherry tomatoes, halved

A drizzle of olive oil

1 tablespoon balsamic vinegar

2 tablespoons chicken stock

Salt and black pepper to the taste

Directions:

1.   Grease your Crockpot with the oil and add bacon on the bottom. Add collard greens, tomatoes, vinegar, stock, salt and pepper, cover and cook on Low for 3 hours.

2.   Divide between plates and serve as a side dish.

3.   Enjoy!

Mustard Greens and Garlic

Ingredients:

2 garlic cloves, minced

1 pound mustard greens, roughly torn

1 tablespoon olive oil

½ cup yellow onion, sliced

Salt and black pepper to the taste

¼ cup veggie stock

¼ teaspoon avocado oil

Directions:

1.   Grease Crockpot with the olive oil, add garlic, greens, onion, salt, pepper and stock, cover and cook on High for 2 hours.

2.   Add avocado oil, toss, divide between plates and serve as a side dish.

3.   Enjoy!

Cheesy Collard Greens

Ingredients:

1 tablespoon jalapeno pepper, chopped

6 eggs, whisked

3 tablespoons olive oil

1 yellow onion, chopped

2 garlic cloves, minced

6 bacon slices, chopped

3 bunches collard greens, chopped

½ cup chicken stock

Salt and black pepper to the taste

1 tablespoon lime juice

1 tablespoon cheddar cheese

Directions:

1.   Add the oil to your Crockpot and arrange jalapeno on the bottom. Add onion, garlic, bacon, collard greens, stock, salt, pepper, lime juice and

whisked eggs, toss, cover and cook on High for 2 hours and 40 minutes.

2.   Add cheese, toss until it melts, divide between plates and serve as a side dish.

3.   Enjoy!

Spring Green Mix

Ingredients:

2 cups mustard greens, chopped

2 cups collard greens, chopped

2 cups veggie stock

1 yellow onion, chopped

Salt and black pepper to the taste

2 tablespoons coconut aminos

2 teaspoons ginger, grated

Directions:

1.   In your Crockpot, mix mustard greens with collard greens, stock, onion, salt, pepper, aminos and ginger, toss, cover and cook on Low for 4 hours.

2.   Divide between plates and serve as a side dish.

3.   Enjoy!

Easy Asparagus

Ingredients:

10 ounces asparagus spears, cut into medium pieces and steamed

Salt and black pepper to the taste

2 tablespoons parmesan, grated

1/3 cup Monterey jack cheese, shredded

2 tablespoons mustard

4 ounces coconut cream

3 tablespoons bacon, cooked and crumbled

Directions:

1.   In your Crockpot, mix asparagus with salt, pepper, mustard, cream and bacon, cover and cook on High for 2 hours and 30 minutes.

2.   Add Monterey jack and parmesan cheese, toss until cheese melts, divide between plates and serve as a side dish.

3.   Enjoy!

Spanish Spinach Mix

Ingredients:

1 yellow onion, sliced

3 tablespoons avocado oil

¼ cup chicken stock

6 garlic cloves, chopped

¼ cup pine nuts, toasted

¼ cup balsamic vinegar

½ teaspoon nutmeg, ground

5 cups mixed spinach and chard

Salt and black pepper to the taste

Directions:

1.   Grease your Crockpot with the oil, add onion, stock, garlic, vinegar, nutmeg, spinach, salt and pepper, toss a bit, cover and cook on High for 3 hours.

2.   Add pine nuts, toss, divide between plates and serve as a side dish.

3.   Enjoy!

Squash and Swiss Chard Mix

Ingredients:

1 red onion, chopped

1 bunch Swiss chard, roughly chopped

1 butternut squash, cubed

1 zucchini, cubed

1 green bell pepper, chopped

Salt and black pepper to the taste

4 cups tomatoes, chopped

1 cup cauliflower florets, chopped

2 cups chicken stock

3 ounces fresh tomato puree

1 pound turkey fillet, chopped

2 garlic cloves, minced

2 teaspoons thyme, chopped

1 teaspoon rosemary, dried

1 tablespoon fennel, minced

½ teaspoon red pepper flake

Directions:

1.   Heat up a pan over medium- high heat, add turkey fillet and garlic, stir and cook until it browns and transfer along with its juices to your Crockpot.

2.   Add onion, Swiss chard, squash, bell pepper, zucchini, tomatoes, cauliflower, fresh tomato puree, stock, thyme, fennel, rosemary, pepper flakes, salt and pepper, stir, cover and cook on High for 2 hours. Divide between plates and serve as a side dish.

3.   Enjoy!

Simple Cherry Tomatoes and Onion Mix

Ingredients:

4 garlic cloves, minced

2 pounds cherry tomatoes, halved

½ red onion, cut into wedges

Salt and black pepper to the taste

3 tablespoons avocado oil

½ teaspoon basil, dried

1 and ½ cups veggie stock

¼ cup parsley, chopped

½ cup goat cheese, crumbled

Directions:

1.   Grease your Crockpot with the oil, add garlic, tomatoes, onion wedges, salt, pepper, basil and stock, cover and cook on Low for 4 hours.

2.   Divide between plates and serve as a side dish with parsley and goat cheese crumbled on top.

3.   Enjoy!

Creamy Eggplant and Tomatoes

Ingredients:

4 tomatoes, cut into wedges

1 teaspoon garlic, minced

¼ yellow onion, chopped

Salt and black pepper to the taste

1 cup chicken stock

1 bay leaf

½ cup coconut cream

2 tablespoons basil, chopped

4 tablespoons parmesan, grated

1 tablespoon olive oil

1 eggplant, cut into medium pieces

Directions:

1.   Grease your Crockpot with the oil, add tomatoes, garlic, onion, salt, pepper, stock, bay leaf,

coconut cream, basil and eggplant, cover and cook on Low for 5 hours.

2.   Add parmesan, toss, divide between plates and serve as a side dish.

3.   Enjoy!

Creamy Radish Mix

Ingredients:

14 ounces radishes, halved

4 tablespoons coconut cream

4 bacon slices, chopped

1 tablespoon green onion, chopped

1 tablespoon cheddar cheese, grated

Salt and black pepper to the taste

Directions:

1.   In your Crockpot, mix radishes with cream, bacon, green onion, salt and pepper, toss, cover and cook on High for 3 hours.

2.   Divide between plates and serve as a side dish with cheese sprinkled on top.

3.   Enjoy!

Keto margarita pizza (V)

Ingredients:

•   2 cups cauliflower florets, blitzed in a food processor until the size of small grains (i.e. couscous)

•   ½ cup tomato passata

•   4 garlic cloves, finely chopped

•   ½ tsp. dried mixed herbs

•   1 tsp. balsamic vinegar or red wine vinegar

•   Salt and pepper

•   5 oz. fresh mozzarella cheese, sliced

•   6 fresh basil leaves

•   1 Tbsp. olive oil

Directions:

1.   Preheat the oven to 375 degrees Fahrenheit and line a baking tray with baking paper

2.	Place the blitzed cauliflower into a bowl and slowly add water as you mix it into a thick, dough-like consistency

3.	Press the cauliflower mixture onto the tray and place it into the oven to pre-cook until lightly golden

4.	Place the tomato passata, garlic, mixed herbs, vinegar, salt, and pepper into a saucepan and place over a medium heat, simmer for about 5 minutes

5.	Spread the passata mixture over the cauliflower base

6.	Place the sliced mozzarella and basil over the pizza base and drizzle with olive oil

7.	Place back into the oven and cook for around 10 minutes until the mozzarella is just beginning to melt

8.	Leave to cool down before slicing and eating

Roasted veggie, halloumi and lemon salad (V)

Ingredients:

•	2 zucchinis, chopped into 1-inch pieces

•	2 cups broccoli florets

- ½ red onion, cut into chunks

- 1 cup butternut pumpkin chunks, (skins removed)

- 3 Tbsp. olive oil

- 8 oz. halloumi cheese, cut into slices

- Finely grated zest of 1 lemon

- Juice of 1 lemon

- Salt and pepper

Directions:

1. Preheat the oven to 375 degrees Fahrenheit and line a baking tray with baking paper

2. Lay the zucchini, broccoli, onion, and butternut pumpkin onto the tray and drizzle over the olive oil, rub the veggies to ensure an even coating of oil

3. Sprinkle the veggies with salt and pepper and pop into the oven to roast for about 25 minutes or until soft and golden

4. While the veggies are roasting, fry the halloumi slices on a hot frying pan until golden on both sides

5.   Place the cooked veggies and halloumi slices into a large bowl and gently toss

6.   Drizzle a little more olive oil over the salad, then add the lemon juice and lemon zest, and finish with salt and pepper to season, toss to combine and coat

7.   Serve warm!

Tempeh Stir-Fry with Cashews and Bok Choy (VG)

Ingredients:

*   1 Tbsp. peanut oil

*   1 tsp. sesame oil

*   8 oz. tempeh, cut into slices or chunks

*   2 Tbsp. soy sauce

*   4 cups bok choy, roughly chopped

*   ¼ cup roasted cashew nuts

*   Fresh cilantro

Directions:

1.   Drizzle both of the oils into a frying pan or wok and place over a high heat

2.   Add the tempeh to the hot oil and turn it with your wooden spoon as it turns golden

3.   Add the bok choy and soy sauce to the hot pan or wok and toss as the bok choy wilts, it should only take a couple of minutes

4.   Serve with a sprinkle of roasted cashews and fresh cilantro!

Creamy Mushroom Cauli-Risotto (V)

Ingredients:

•   2 Tbsp. olive oil

•   6 garlic cloves, finely chopped

•   ½ onion, finely chopped

•   ½ cup dry white wine

•   2 cups sliced brown mushrooms

•   6 cups cauliflower, blitzed in a food processor until the size of rice

•   3 cups vegetable stock

•   2 Tbsp. butter

•   ¼ cup grated Parmesan cheese

- Salt and pepper

Directions:

1.   Drizzle the olive oil into a large frying pan or pot and place over a medium heat

2.   Add the garlic and onion to the hot pot and stir as the onion softens

3.   Add the wine to the pot and stir as the alcohol evaporates

4.   Add the mushrooms and cauliflower to the pot and stir as they cook and soften

5.   Slowly add the vegetable stock in increments of about ⅓ cup and allow it to reduce slightly before adding the next lot, repeat until all of the stock has been added and the risotto is creamy

6.   Stir in the butter, Parmesan, salt and pepper and place the lid onto the pan or pot and leave for about 5 minutes to let everything meld together

7.   Stir the risotto before serving with a sprinkle of fresh herbs for color

Broccoli and Parmesan Soup (V)

Ingredients:

- 2 Tbsp. olive oil

- 1 onion, roughly chopped

- 4 garlic cloves, finely chopped

- 6 cups broccoli florets

- 4 cups vegetable stock

- ½ cup grated Parmesan cheese

- ⅓ cup mascarpone cheese

- Salt and pepper

Directions:

1. Add the olive oil to a large pot and place over a medium heat

2. Add the onion and garlic to the pot and stir as the onions soften

3. Add the broccoli and stock to the pot and place the lid on to allow to come to a boil

4. Once the broccoli is nice and soft, leave it to cool slightly before using a hand-held stick blender to blitz until smooth

5.   Add the parmesan to the pot and stir as it melts into the soup

6.   Stir the mascarpone, salt, and pepper into the soup and serve right away!

Zoodles with Pesto Sauce (V)

Ingredients:

*   6 zucchinis, cut into noodles with a spiralizer

*   4 Tbsp. pesto (store bought is totally fine)

*   1/3 cup finely grated Parmesan

*   1 Tbsp. olive oil

Directions:

1.   Bring a pot of water to a boil, add lots of salt, and add the zoodles, cook for about 1 minute (they don't need long at all! Just a little while to take away the raw taste)

2.   Drain the zoodles and add the pesto, parmesan and olive oil, toss to coat the zoodles

3.   Serve right away!

Green Curry with Tofu and Sugar Snap Peas (VG)

Ingredients:

•   4 Tbsp. vegan green curry paste (store bought is fine as long as it's vegan friendly)

•   12 oz. firm tofu, cut into cubes

•   1 ½ cups sugar snap peas

•   1 cup button mushrooms, sliced

•   1 ½ cups coconut cream

•   1 cup vegetable stock

Directions:

1.   Place a large frying pan or pot over a medium-high heat

2.   Add the curry paste to the pot and heat until fragrant, (about 2 minutes)

3.   Add the tofu and stir to coat in curry paste, allow to cook for about 2 minutes

4.   Stir in the sugar snap peas and mushrooms and allow them to cook for about 2 minutes

5.   Pour the coconut cream and vegetable stock into the pot, stir to combine, and allow to simmer for about 5 minutes

6.   Serve alone or with cauliflower rice!

Creamy Asparagus Soup (VG)

Ingredients:

*   2 Tbsp. olive oil

*   1 onion, finely chopped

*   4 garlic cloves, finely chopped

*   40 asparagus spears (about 4 bunches), roughly chopped

*   2 cups vegetable stock

*   1 cup coconut cream

*   Salt and pepper

Directions:

1.   Pour the olive oil into a large pot and place over a high heat

2.   Add the onions, garlic, and asparagus and stir as they soften, about 3 minutes

3.   Add the vegetable stock, coconut cream, salt and pepper, stir to combine

4.   Pop the lid onto the pot and allow to simmer until the asparagus is nice and soft

5.   Allow to cool slightly before using a hand-held blender to blitz until smooth

Fried Eggplant with Soy-Lime Sauce (VG)

Ingredients:

•   3 Tbsp. olive oil

•   2 eggplants, cut into 1-inch slices

•   Salt and pepper

•   3 Tbsp. soy sauce

•   1 tsp. sesame oil

•   Juice of 1 lime

•   ½ fresh red chili, finely chopped

Directions:

1.   Drizzle the olive oil into a non-stick frying pan and place over a medium-high heat

2.   Add the eggplant slices to the hot oil and sprinkle with salt and pepper

3.   Cook the eggplant slices on both sides until nice and golden before taking them off the heat and placing onto a serving plate

4.   Drizzle the soy sauce, sesame oil, and lime juice over the cooked tofu and sprinkle the fresh red chili over the top

5.   Serve right away!

Cabbage, Apple, and Tofu Salad (VG)

Ingredients:

•   4 cups shredded cabbage

•   2 cups shredded iceberg lettuce

•   1 crispy apple, grated

•   10 oz. firm tofu, cut into 1-inch slices

•   1 tsp. sesame oil

•   1 Tbsp. avocado oil

•   2 Tbsp. soy sauce

•   2 Tbsp. toasted sesame seeds

Directions:

1.   Place the shredded cabbage, lettuce, and apple into a large salad bowl and toss to combine

2.   Drizzle the sesame and olive oils into a non-stick frying pan and place over a high heat

3.   Add the tofu to the hot oil and fry on both sides until golden

4.   Add the soy sauce and sesame seeds to the tofu and toss to coat

5.   Add the cooked tofu and sesame seeds to the salad and toss to combine

6.   Had an extra drizzle of avocado oil over the salad before serving!

Spicy Roasted Brussels Sprouts with Coconut Peanut Sauce (VG)

Ingredients:

•   12 Brussels sprouts, cut in half

•   2 Tbsp. olive oil

•   Fresh red chili, finely chopped

•   Salt and pepper

Sauce:

- ¾ cup coconut cream

- 4 Tbsp. crunchy peanut butter

- ½ tsp. sesame oil

- 1 Tbsp. soy sauce

Directions:

1.   Preheat the oven to 400 degrees Fahrenheit and line a baking tray with baking paper

2.   Lay the Brussels sprouts onto the tray and rub with olive oil, chili, salt, and pepper until coated

3.   Roast the Brussels sprouts until golden and just soft but not mushy

4.   While the sprouts roast, make the sauce: place the coconut cream, peanut butter, sesame oil, and soy sauce into a small pot and place over a low-medium heat. Stir as the sauce simmers and melts together

5.   Pop the cooked Brussels sprouts onto a serving plate and either pour the sauce over them, or place it into a small bowl so you and your guests can dip the sprouts into it at your leisure

Chapter 12: Ketogenic Snacks & Dessert

Egg Float with Herbs

Ingredients

- 2 tbs organic butter, pastured

- 1 tbs coconut oil

- 2 garlic cloves, peeled and finely chopped

- 1 tsp fresh thyme leaves

- ½ cup fresh cilantro, chopped

- ½ cup fresh parsley, chopped

- 4 organic eggs (pastured

- ¼ tsp ground cumin

- ¼ tsp ground cayenne

- ½ tsp sea salt

Directions

1.   Melt butter in a skillet (preferably non-stick along with coconut oil.

2.　　　Add garlic and cook till it starts to turn brown.

3.　　　Mix in thyme and cook for another half a minute or so. Avoid the garlic from getting burnt.

4.　　　Add the fresh chopped cilantro and parsley. Mix well and cook till it becomes crispy.

5.　　　Reduce the heat and break the eggs directly in the pan (keeping the yolk intact.

6.　　　Let it cook for 5 minutes on reduced flame till the yolks look set, yet soft from within.

7.　　　Remove from the pan and serve hot. (Goes well with any sausage of your choice.

Hazelnut and Lime Pie

Ingredients

For the Crust

- 2 cups raw hazelnuts, grinded
- 4 Tbs Chia seeds
- 1Tbs Swerve
- 4 Tbs organic butter, melted
- 1 egg
- 1 Tbs coconut oil

For the Filling

- 1.5 cup coconut cream
- 1.5 cup sour cream
- 3 large eggs
- 1 cup fresh key lime juice
- 3 Tbs Swerve
- 1 Tbs Key Lime Zest
- ½ cup unsweetened coconut shavings

Directions

1. Set the oven to preheat at 375° F
2. Take the hazelnuts and grind them till they become floury. Add chia seeds, sweetener (Swerve and melted butter. Mix them well to form dough.
3. Take a 6x9 sized baking dish and grease it with coconut oil.
4. Lay the crust over it and press to flatten it. Place it in the oven and let it bake for 15-20 minutes.
5. To prepare the filling –
6. Take a mixing bowl and pour in the coconut cream along with sour cream and blend them well. Add in the eggs, some lime juice, swerve, some lime zest and coconut shavings.
7. Blend them well so as to form a smooth froth.

8. Once the crust is baked, pour the prepared filling over it and spread it evenly.
9. Place it in the oven again and let it bake for around 40-45 minutes at 350°
10. Once done, take it out of the oven and let it cool. Sprinkle some coconut flakes over it once it has cooled and place it in the refrigerator to rest, preferably overnight.

Cacao and Chia Pudding

Ingredients

- 2 tbs traditional herbal coffee blend

- ⅓ cup coconut cream - undiluted

- 1 tbs organic vanilla extract

- 1 tbs Swerve

- 2 tbs (15 gr Cacao nibs

- ⅓ cup dry chia seeds

Directions

1.   Take the coffee blend and pour in some hot water in it (Around 2 cups.

2.   Brew it for around 15-20 minutes till the water volume reduces to half.

3.   Strain it and blend it with coconut cream, swerve and a bit of vanilla extract.

4.   Add to it the cacao nibs and the chia seeds. Mix it all well to combine the ingredients.

5.   Pour the mixture in serving glasses and refrigerate for around half an hour or so.

6.   Garnish with some cacao nibs and serve.

Frozen Coconut and Pecan Rollers

Ingredients

- 2 Cups Raw Pecans

- 1 Cup Grated or Shredded Coconut

- 2 Oz Unsweetened baking Chocolate

- 3 Tbs Swerve or 1 Tsp Green Stevia

- 1 Tbs Vanilla Extract

Directions

1.	Take a food process jar and put in the raw pecans, shredded coconut along with the baking chocolate.

2.	Blend it well for few seconds.

3.	Add in the Stevia and vanilla extract and blend it again to form dough.

4.	Take the dough out on a parchment sheet and roll it. Place it in the chiller for it to rest for around 2-3 hours.

5.	Once it is set, take it out from the chiller and cut ½ inch sized slices out of it.

6.	Serve chilled. Store in the chiller when not serving.

Hazelnut and cocoa candies

Ingredients

For the Filling:

•	2 ounces / 56 grams cocoa butter

•	2 to 3 tablespoons Swerve - powdered in the grinder

•	1 ounce / 28 grams unsweetened cocoa powder

- 2 ounces / 56 grams toasted hazelnuts

- 12 whole hazelnuts

For the coating -

- 1.5 ounces / 42 grams cocoa butter

- 0.5 ounce / 14 grams unsweetened cocoa powder

- 1 tablespoon Swerve , grin

Directions

1. Take a saucepan (preferably double-boiler and melt some cocoa butter in it.

2. As the butter melts, add the cocoa powder and swerve and mix well.

3. Using a grinder or a food processor, grind the hazelnuts and add it to the butter and cocoa mixture.

4. Mix well until a smooth paste is formed.

5. Prepare a water bath and add some ice in it (in order to fasten the cooling and place this saucepan in it. Prevent the water from entering the pan.

6.   Keep stirring till the mixture becomes hard enough. Prepare 12 balls out of it and place a single hazelnut on top of each ball.

Arrange these balls on a cookie sheet covered with a parchment sheet and let it rest in the chiller for a around 15-20 minutes.

To prepare the coating –

7.   Take a medium sized pan and melt the cocoa butter in it. Add the cocoa powder and swerve and beat it well.

8.   Cook it till it reaches the liquid state and then remove it from flame. Keep it aside to let it cool till it starts thickening

9.   Check the balls inside the chiller and take them out if they have become solid enough.

10.   Pierce a tooth-pick slightly inside each ball and then dip it in the prepared coating. Roll them well so that they are completely coated.

11.   Place them in the refrigerator till coating becomes hard and take them off the tooth-pick.

12.   Note – To thicken the chocolate coating, double the quantity of ingredients used to prepare the coating and again coat the balls in it.

Banana and Hazelnut Gelato

Ingredients

- 3 organic bananas peeled, cut in rounds and frozen.

- 1 cup toasted hazelnuts, grinded

- ¼ cup dark cacao powder

- 1 tablespoon liquid organic vanilla

Directions

1. Remove the frozen bananas from the freezer when you are about to start preparing..

2. Make sure the toasted hazelnuts are grinded well and are floury.

3. Take a blender and add the bananas, grounded hazelnut flour, cacao powder and liquid vanilla to it. Blend them together till they forma a smooth paste.

4. Take out the prepared gelato in a large serving bowl and place it in the freezer.

5. Serve chilled garnished with a single hazelnut piece on top.

6. Note – Store it frozen but take it out from the freezer at least half an hour before serving.

Slow Cooker Chicken Gizzards

Ingredients

- 1 bunch of organic cilantro, washed and cleaned from stems

- 3 large cloves of organic garlic, peeled and sliced

- 1 small organic onion

- 1 pound of free range chicken gizzards

- ¼ cup Passata di Pomodoro

- ½ cup white wine

- ¼ cup water

- a good pinch of Celtic sea salt

Directions

1. Mix all the ingredients in a slow cooker and arrange the water levels so that the chicken gizzards are submerged half way.

2.   Let it cook for around 5-6 hours.

3.   Once the chicken is cooked thoroughly, remove from heat and serve hot.

Stuffed Parmesan and Pepper Jack Pinwheels

Ingredients

For the crust

- 1Tbs lard

- 1 Tbs butter

- ½ cup water

- ½ Tsp sea salt

- ¾ cups coconut flour

- 2 tbs Psyllium husk

- 1 pastured egg, beaten

For the filling:

- ½ cup parmesan cheese, grated

- 150 gr pepper jack cheese, shredded

- freshly ground black pepper to taste

Directions

To prepare the crust –

1.   Melt some butter in a saucepan and add lard to it.

2.   After couple of minutes, pour some water in it and keep stirring. Prevent it from boiling.

3.   Take a mixing bowl and combine the coconut flour, husk and some salt (as per taste in it. Mix them well.

4.   Add the egg and beat it well. Avoid forming lumps.

5.   Gently pour in the hot water with butter and whisk it to form dough. Keep it aside and let it rest.

To prepare the filling –

6.   Set the oven to preheat at 350° F

7.   Mix the parmesan with pepper jack cheese and add the grounded black pepper.

8.   Once the dough has rested for a while, shape it into a ball.

9.   Cut a parchment paper into two halves and place the dough ball in between them.

10.   Roll the ball (1/4 inch in thickness from over the parchment sheet and then remove it.

Evenly spread the cheese mixture over the dough and then roll the dough from one end to the other in such a way that the cheese remains in the center.

11.   Squeeze the ends of the dough together to close it.

12.   Cut slices from this roll of around ¼ inch thickness.

13.   Arrange the slices on a cookie sheet (greased and place it on the oven to bake for around 15-20 minutes.

14.   Once done, let them cool and then remove them from the sheet.

Peanut Butter Mousse

Ingredients:

•   ½ can coconut cream

•   4 tbsps. peanut butter, unsweetened

•   1 tsp. stevia

Directions:

1.   Combine all ingredients and whip for one minute, until mixture forms peaks.

2.   Chill for at least three hours, or until a mousse texture is achieved.

Nutritional Information: 206 Calories, 18g Fats, 6g Net Carbs, and 5g Protein.

Almond butter balls

Ingredients:

- 3 tbsps. almond butter

- 3 tbsps. carob powder

- 3 tsps. almond flour

- 2 tsps. powdered Yacon powder

- ½ c. coconut flakes, unsweetened

Directions:

1.   In a bowl, combine almond butter, carob powder, almond flour, and Erythritol.

2.   Stir until combined.

3.   Place coconut flakes in a small bowl.

4.   Scoop prepared a mixture with a small ice cream scoop and drop into coconut flakes.

5.   Roll until completely covered with the coconut flakes. Arrange the balls on a plate and refrigerate for 4-6 hour or until firm.

6.   Serve and enjoy.

Peanut Butter Cookies

Ingredients:

•   1 c. smooth peanut butter

•   ¾ c. almond flour

•   ½ c. powdered Erythritol

•   ¼ c. almond milk

•   1 scoop hemp protein powder, vanilla flavored

•   1 tsp. baking soda

Directions:

1.   Heat oven to 350F and line a baking sheet with baking paper.

2.   In a bowl, cream peanut butter, and powdered Erythritol.

3.   In a separate bowl, combine all dry ingredients.

4.   Fold the dry ingredients into peanut butter and stir until you have a crumbly mix.

5.   Stir in almond milk and roll dough into balls (2 tablespoons per cookie).

6.   Drop dough onto baking sheet and flatten with a fork, making a crisscross pattern.

7.   Bake cookies 10 minutes. Cool completely before serving.

Stuffed Apples

Ingredients:

*   4 cored green apple

*   ½ c. melted coconut butter

*   ¼ c. almond butter, unsweetened

*   2 tbsps. Cinnamon, ground

*   Ground nutmeg

*   Salt

- 4 tbsps. Shredded and unsweetened coconut

- 1 c. water

Directions:

1.   In a bowl, mix together coconut butter, almond butter, cinnamon, nutmeg, and salt.

2.   Arrange the apples in a slow cooker and place the water in the bottom. With a spoon, place butter mixture into each apple evenly. Top each apple with shredded coconut.

3.   Set the slow cooker on Low. Cover and cook for about 2-3 hours.

4.   Serve warm.

Berry Crumble

Ingredients:

- 1 c. almond flour

- 2 tbsps. melted butter

- 1 tbsp. applesauce, unsweetened

- 4 c. fresh mixed berries

- 1 tbsp. chopped butter

Directions:

1.   In a bowl, add flour, melted butter, and applesauce and mix until crumbly mixture forms.

2.   In the bottom of a slow cooker, place the berries and dot with chopped butter. Sprinkle the topping mixture over the berries evenly.

3.   Set the slow cooker on Low. Cover and cook for about 2 hours.

4.   Unplug the slow cooker and let the crumble cool slightly. Cut into desired pieces and serve warm.

Cocoa Pumpkin Fudge

Ingredients:

*   1 c. organic unsweetened pumpkin puree

*   1¾ c. cocoa butter

*   1 tsp. allspice

*   1 tbsp. coconut oil, melted

Directions:

1.   Line 8-inch glass dish with baking paper.

2.   Melt cocoa butter over medium heat.

3.   Stir in pumpkin puree and allspice. Stir to combine.

4.   Add coconut oil and stir well. Transfer the mixture into a prepared glass dish and press down to distribute evenly.

5.   Cover with a second piece of baking paper and refrigerate 2 hours.

6.   Slice and serve.

Blackberry cheesecake smoothie

Ingredients:

• 6 Ice cubes

• Sweetener

• ¾ c. Coconut milk

• ¼ tsp. Vanilla extract

• 1 tsp. Coconut oil

• ¼ c. frozen blackberries

• ¼ c. Water

Directions:

1.   Cream the coconut milk: This is a simple process. All you need to do is place the can of coconut milk in the refrigerator overnight. The next morning, open the can and spoon out the coconut milk that has solidified. Don't shake the can before opening. Discard the liquids.

2.   Add all of the ingredients, save the ice cubes, to the blender and blend on low speed until pureed. Thin with water as needed.

3.   Add in the ice cubes and blend until the smoothie reaches your desired consistency.

Orangesicle smoothie

Ingredients:

•   6 Ice cubes

•   Sweetener

•   ¾ c. Coconut milk

•   1 scoop Vanilla whey protein

•   2 tbsps. Coconut oil

•   2 oz. Plain skyr

•   8 oz. Fresh orange juice

•   2 oz. shredded Carrot

- 1 ripe Mango

Directions:

1.   Cream the coconut milk: This is a simple process. All you need to do is place the can of coconut milk in the refrigerator overnight. The next morning, open the can and spoon out the coconut milk that has solidified. Don't shake the can before opening. Discard the liquids.

2.   Add all of the ingredients, save the ice cubes, to the blender and blend on low speed until pureed. Thin with water as needed.

3.   Add in the ice cubes and blend until the smoothie reaches your desired consistency.

Vanilla ice cream smoothie

Ingredients:

- 6 Ice cubes

- Sweetener

- ¼ c. Mascarpone

- 2 Egg yolk

- 1 tbsp. Coconut oil

- ¼ tsp. Vanilla extract

- 1 oz. Whipped topping

Directions:

1.   Add all of the ingredients, save the ice cubes, to the blender and blend on low speed until pureed. Thin with water as needed.

2.   Add in the ice cubes and blend until the smoothie reaches your desired consistency.

3.   Top with whipped topping prior to serving.

Strawberry rhubarb pie smoothie

Ingredients:

- 6 Ice cubes

- Sweetener

- ¾ c. Coconut milk

- 5 tsps. Powdered Ginger

- ¼ tsp. Vanilla extract

- 2 tbsps. Almond butter

- 2 Rhubarb stalks

- 1.4 oz. Strawberries

- 1 Organic egg

- ¼ tsp. Vanilla extract

- 5 grated Ginger root

Directions:

1.   Cream the coconut milk: This is a simple process. All you need to do is place the can of coconut milk in the refrigerator overnight. The next morning, open the can and spoon out the coconut milk that has solidified. Don't shake the can before opening. Discard the liquids.

2.   Add all of the ingredients, save the ice cubes, to the blender and blend on low speed until pureed. Thin with water as needed.

3.   Add in the ice cubes and blend until the smoothie reaches your desired consistency.

Avocado Pudding

Ingredients:

- 2 pitted and chopped avocados

- 2 tsps. vanilla extract

- 8 drops stevia

- 1 tbsp. lime juice

- 14 oz. coconut milk

- 1½ c. water

Directions:

1.   In your instant pot, mix avocado with coconut milk, vanilla extract, stevia and lime juice, blend well and divide into 4 ramekins.

2.   Add the water to your instant pot, add the steamer basket, add ramekins inside, cover and cook on High for 2 minutes.

3.   Keep puddings in the fridge until you serve them.

4.   Enjoy!

Orange Cake

Ingredients:

- 6 large eggs

- 1 quartered orange

- 1½ c. water

- 1 tsp. vanilla extract

- 1 tsp. baking powder

- 9 oz. almond meal

- 4 tbsps. swerve

- 2 tbsps. grated orange zest

- 2 oz. stevia

- 4 oz. cream cheese

- 4 oz. coconut yogurt

Directions:

1. In your food processor, mix orange with almond meal, swerve, eggs, baking powder, and vanilla extract, pulse well and transfer to a cake pan.

2. Add the water to your instant pot, add steamer basket, add cake pan inside, cover and cook on High for 25 minutes.

3. In a bowl, mix cream cheese with orange zest, coconut yogurt, and stevia and stir well.

4. Spread this well over cake, slice and serve it.

5. Enjoy!

Icy Pops

Ingredients:

- 1 peeled and pitted avocado

- 1½ tsps. vanilla paste

- 1 c. coconut milk

- 2 tbsps. almond butter

- Drops of stevia

- ¼ tsp. Ceylon cinnamon

Directions:

1. Combine all ingredients in a food blender.

2. Blend until smooth.

3. Transfer the mixture into popsicle molds and insert popsicle sticks.

4. Freeze 4 hours or until firm.

5. Serve.

Spicy Mango Dip

Ingredients:

- 1 chopped shallot

- 1 tbsp. coconut oil

- ¼ tsp. cardamom powder

- 2 tbsps. minced ginger

- ½ tsp. cinnamon powder

- 2 chopped mangos

- 2 chopped red hot chilies

- 1 chopped apple

- ¼ c. raisins

- 5 tbsps. stevia

- 1¼ apple cider vinegar

Directions:

1.   Set your instant pot on Sauté mode, add oil, heat it up, add shallot and ginger, stir and cook for 3 minutes.

2.   Add cinnamon, hot peppers, cardamom, mangos, apple, raisins, stevia, and cider, stir, cover and cook on High for 7 minutes.

3.   Set the pot on simmer mode, cook your dip for 6 minutes more, transfer to bowls and serve cold as a snack.

4.   Enjoy!

Cranberry Dip

Ingredients:

•   2½ tsps. grated lemon zest

•   3 tbsps. lemon juice

•   12 oz. cranberries

•   4 tbsps. stevia

Directions:

1.   In your instant pot, mix lemon juice with stevia, lemon zest, and cranberries, stir, cover and cook on High for 2 minutes.

2.   Set the pot on simmer mode, stir your dip for a couple more minutes, transfer to a bowl and serve with some biscuits as a snack.

3.   Enjoy!

Chapter 13: Ketogenic Vegetables

Cheesy and Buttery Pork Chops

Ingredients

1/2 stick butter, room temperature

1/2 cup white onion, chopped

4 ounces button mushrooms, sliced

1/3 pound pork loin chops

1 teaspoon dried parsley flakes

Salt and ground black pepper, to taste

1/2 cup Swiss cheese, shredded

Directions

1.   Melt 1/4 of the butter stick in a skillet over medium heat. Then, sauté the onions and mushrooms until the onions are translucent and the mushrooms are tender and fragrant, about 5 minutes. Reserve.

2.   Then, melt the remaining 1/4 of the butter stick and cook pork until slightly browned on all sides, about 10 minutes.

3.   Add the onion mixture, parsley, salt, and pepper. Lastly, top with cheese; cover and let it cook on medium-low heat until cheese has melted.

4.   Serve immediately and enjoy!

Filipino Nilaga Soup

Ingredients

1 teaspoon butter

1 pound pork ribs, boneless and cut into small pieces

1 shallot, chopped

2 garlic cloves, minced

1 (1/2-inch piece fresh ginger, chopped

1 cup water

2 cups chicken stock

1 tablespoon patis (fish sauce

1 cup fresh tomatoes, pureed

1 cup cauliflower "rice"

Sea salt and ground black pepper, to taste

Directions

1.   Melt the butter in a pot over medium-high heat. Then, cook the pork ribs on all sides for 5 to 6 minutes.

2.   Add the shallot, garlic and ginger; cook an additional 3 minutes. Add the remaining ingredients.

3.   Let it cook, covered, for 30 to 35 minutes. Ladle into individual bowls and serve.

Pork Tenderloin with Southern Cabbage

Ingredients

The Pork tenderloin:

1/2 pound pork tenderloin

Celtic sea salt and freshly cracked black pepper, to taste

1/2 teaspoon granulated garlic

1/4 teaspoon ginger powder

1/2 teaspoon dried sage

1 tablespoon lard, room temperature

The Cabbage:

4 ounces cabbage, sliced into strips

1/3 cup vegetable broth

2 tablespoons sherry wine

1/2 teaspoon mustard seeds

Celtic sea salt, to taste

1/2 teaspoon black peppercorns

Directions

1.   Season the pork with salt, black pepper, granulated garlic, ginger powder, and sage.

2.   Melt the lard in a pan over moderate heat. Sear the pork for 7 to 8 minutes, turning periodically.

3.   In a pan that is preheated over medium heat, bring the cabbage, broth, sherry, and mustard seeds to a boil over high heat.

4.   Season with salt and black peppercorns; cook, stirring periodically, until the cabbage is tender, about 12 minutes; do not overcook.

5.   Serve the pork with sautéed cabbage on the side. Enjoy!

Indian-Style Fried Pork

Ingredients

1 teaspoon shallot powder

1 teaspoon porcini powder

1 teaspoon garlic powder

1/2 teaspoon cumin

1/4 teaspoon turmeric powder

1 cinnamon stick

2 dried Kashmiri red chillies, roasted

Sea salt and ground black pepper, to taste

1 pound pork shoulder

1/2 cup ground pork rinds

1/2 cup Parmesan cheese, grated

2 eggs

2 tablespoons tallow

Directions

1.   Blend the spices together with the cinnamon and chillies until you have a smooth paste. Rub this paste all over the pork shoulder.

2.   In a bowl, combine the pork rinds with parmesan cheese. In a separate bowl, whisk the eggs.

3.   Slice the pork into small pieces; dip the pork in the egg and then, cover it with the pork rind mixture.

4.   Melt the tallow in a skillet over medium-high heat. Cook the pork for 2 to 3 minutes per side. Enjoy!

Italian-Style Spicy Meatballs

Ingredients

Sauce:

3 ounces Asiago cheese, grated

1⁄4 cup mayonnaise

1 chili pepper, minced

1 teaspoon yellow mustard

1 teaspoon Italian parsley

1/2 teaspoon red pepper flakes, crushed

1/2 teaspoon sea salt

1/2 teaspoon ground black pepper

Meatballs:

1/2 pound ground beef

1 egg

1 tablespoon olive oil

Directions

1.   In a bowl, thoroughly combine the cheese, mayo, chili, mustard, parsley, red pepper, salt, and black pepper.

2.   Then, stir in the ground beef and egg. Stir to combine well. Shape the mixture into meatballs.

3.　　　Now, heat the oil in a skillet over a moderate flame. Once hot, cook the meatballs for 2 to 3 minutes on each side. Serve and enjoy!

Rich Double-Cheese Meatloaf

Ingredients

2 teaspoons sunflower oil

1/2 cup onions, chopped

2 cloves garlic, minced

1 bell pepper, seeded and chopped

1 jalapeno pepper, seeded and chopped

3/4 pound ground beef

1/4 pound bacon, chopped

1/2 Swiss cheese, grated

1/2 cup Parmesan cheese, grated

1 egg, whisked

1 teaspoon oyster sauce

Sea salt and ground black pepper, to taste

1 ripe tomato, pureed

1 teaspoon Dijon mustard

Directions

1.   Start by preheating your oven to 390 degrees F. Lightly grease a baking pan with a nonstick cooking spray.

2.   Heat the oil in a pan over a moderate flame. Now, sauté the onions, garlic, and peppers until tender and aromatic, about 5 minutes.

3.   In a mixing bowl, thoroughly combine the ground beef, bacon, cheese, egg, oyster sauce, salt, and ground black pepper. Form the mixture into a loaf and press it into the baking pan; spread the mixture of pureed tomato and mustard over the top.

4.   Cover the dish with foil and bake for 50 minutes in the preheated oven. Enjoy!

Meat and Goat Cheese Stuffed Mushrooms

Ingredients

4 ounces ground beef

2 ounces ground pork

Kosher salt and ground black pepper, to taste

1/4 cup goat cheese, crumbled

2 tablespoons Romano cheese, grated

2 tablespoons shallot, minced

1 garlic clove, minced

1 teaspoon dried basil

1/2 teaspoon dried oregano

1/2 teaspoon dried rosemary

20 button mushrooms, stems removed

Direction

1.   Combine all ingredients, except for the mushrooms, in a mixing bowl. Then, stuff the mushrooms with this filling.

2.   Bake in the preheated oven at 370 degrees F approximately 18 minutes. Serve warm or cold. Enjoy!

Shredded Beef with Herbs

Ingredients

1 tablespoon olive oil

1 pound rib eye, cut into strips

2 tablespoons rice wine

1/4 cup beef bone broth

Sea salt and ground black pepper, to taste

2 tablespoons fresh parsley, finely chopped

2 tablespoons fresh chives, finely chopped

2 chipotle peppers in adobo sauce, chopped

1 garlic clove, crushed

2 small-sized ripe tomatoes, pureed

1 yellow onion, peeled and chopped

1/2 teaspoon dry mustard

1 teaspoon dried basil

1 teaspoon dried marjoram

Directions

1.   Heat the oil in a pan over medium-high heat. Sear the beef for 6 to 7 minutes, stirring periodically. Work in batches.

2.   Add the remaining ingredients, reduce the heat to medium-low and let it cook for 40 minutes.

3.   Shred the beef and serve. Enjoy!

Chinese Ground Beef Skillet

Ingredients

1 tablespoon sesame oil

1/2 pound ground chuck

1 shallot, minced

1 garlic clove, minced

1 (1/2-inch piece ginger root, peeled and grated

1 bell pepper, seeded and sliced

4 ounces brown mushrooms, sliced

1 teaspoon tamari soy sauce

1 tablespoon rice wine

2 whole star anise

Himalayan salt and ground black pepper, to taste

Directions

1.   Heat the oil in a pan over a moderate flame. Now, cook the ground chuck until it is no longer pink. Reserve.

2.   Then, cook the shallot, garlic, ginger, pepper, and mushrooms in pan drippings. Add the remaining ingredients along with reserved beef to the pan.

3.   Reduce the heat to medium-low; let it simmer for 2 to 3 minutes longer. Make sure to stir continuously. Enjoy!

Easy Steak Salad

Ingredients

2 tablespoons olive oil

8 ounces flank steak, salt-and-pepper-seasoned

1 cucumber, sliced

1/2 cup onions, finely sliced

1 ripe avocado, peeled and sliced

2 medium-sized heirloom tomatoes, sliced

2 ounces baby arugula

1 tablespoon fresh coriander, chopped

3 tablespoons lime juice

Directions

1.   Heat 1 tablespoon of olive oil in a pan over medium-high heat. Cook the flank steak for 5 minutes, turning once or twice.

2.   Let stand for 10 minutes; then, slice thinly across the grain. Transfer the meat to a bowl.

3.   Add cucumbers, shallots, avocado, tomatoes, baby arugula, and fresh coriander. Now, drizzle your salad with lime juice and the remaining 1 tablespoon of olive oil.

4.   Serve well chilled and enjoy!

Saucy Skirt Steak with Broccoli

Ingredients

1/2 pound skirt steak, sliced into pieces

2 tablespoons butter, room temperature

1/2 pound broccoli, cut into florets

1/2 cup scallions, chopped

1 clove garlic, pressed

Marinade:

1/2 teaspoon ground black pepper

1 teaspoon red pepper flakes

1/2 teaspoon sea salt

2 tablespoons olive oil

1 tablespoon tamari sauce

1/4 cup wine vinegar

Directions

1.   In a ceramic bowl, thoroughly combine all ingredients for the marinade. Add the beef and allow it to sit in your refrigerator for 2 hours.

2.   Melt 1 tablespoon of butter in a skillet over high to medium-high heat. Cook the broccoli for 2 minutes, stirring frequently, until it is tender but bright green. Reserve.

3.   Melt the remaining tablespoon of butter in the skillet. Once hot, cook the scallions and garlic until aromatic, about 2 minutes. Reserve.

4.   Next, sear the beef, adding a small amount of the marinade. Cook until well browned on all sides or about 10 minutes.

5.   Add the reserved vegetables and cook for a few minutes more or until everything is heated through. Enjoy!

Chapter 14: Poultry

Honey Barbecue Chicken Wings

Ingredients:

2 lbs. chicken wings

½ cup water

2 teaspoons paprika

1 teaspoon red pepper flakes

½ cup apple juice

Cayenne pepper

¾ cup honey barbecue sauce

Sea salt and black pepper to taste

1 teaspoon Truvia

½ teaspoon basil, dried

Directions:

1.   Place the chicken wings into your instant pot.

2.   Add the barbecue sauce, salt, pepper, paprika, red pepper, Truvia, water, and apple juice. Stir, cover and cook on the Poultry setting for 10minutes.

3.   Release the pressure naturally for 10minutes.

4.   Transfer the chicken wings to a baking sheet, add the sauce, place under preheated broiler for 7minutes.

5.   Turn chicken wings over and broil for an additional 7minutes.

6.   Divide among serving plates. Serve hot!

Sticky Chicken Drumsticks

Ingredients:

8 chicken drumsticks

1 teaspoon ginger, fresh, grated

3 garlic cloves, finely chopped

3 tablespoons olive oil

Juice of 1 lemon

2 tablespoons soy sauce

Directions:

1.   Mix the lemon juice, olive oil, ginger, garlic, and soy sauce in your instant pot. Add the chicken drumsticks and stir to coat them.

2.   Secure the instant pot lid and set it to the Poultry setting for a Preparation Time of 20minutes.

3.   Release the pressure naturally for 15minutes.

4.   Divide drumsticks on to serving plates, and drizzle sauce over them. Serve hot!

Chicken, Broccoli, & Cheese

Ingredients:

20ounces chicken breast,

cooked, shredded

1 teaspoon oregano, dried

½ teaspoon paprika

1ounce pork rinds

1 cup cheddar cheese, shredded

½ cup heavy cream

½ cup sour cream

2 cups broccoli, florets

2 tablespoons olive oil

Directions:

1.   Place the cooked, shredded chicken into your instant pot. In a bowl mix broccoli, olive oil, and sour cream.

2.   Pour over chicken and stir. Pour heavy cream over top and season. On Manual setting cook on low for 40minutes.

3.   Release the pressure naturally for 15minutes. Crush the pork rinds.

4.   Add the pork rinds and cheese on top of mixture, cover with lid and cook for an additional 5minutes.

5.   Divide among serving dishes. Serve warm!

Instant Pot Cream Chicken & Sausage

Ingredients:

1 ½ lbs. chicken breasts, boneless, skinless, cut into strips

1 large Italian sausage, sliced

18 ounce package of cream cheese

2 tablespoons grainy mustard

1 small yellow onion, diced

½ cup white wine

1 cup chicken stock

Scallions, chopped for garnish

Salt and black pepper to taste

2 tablespoons coconut oil

Directions:

1.   Set your instant pot to the sautė mode, add the oil and heat. Add the sausage, and chicken breast strips, and brown for about 5minutes.

2.   Add the yellow onion, and cook for an additional 3minutes and stir. In a mixing bowl combine the cheese, mustard, stock, wine, garlic, salt and pepper.

3.   Pour the cheese mix over the chicken and sausage mix, and stir to combine. Place the lid onto your instant pot and set it on Poultry setting for 40minutes.

4.   Release the pressure naturally for 10minutes. Stir mix and serve over a bed of cauliflower rice or zucchini pasta. Serve warm!

Instant Pot Chicken Hash

Ingredients:

1 lb. chicken, boneless, skinless, diced

2 cups chicken stock

1 cup sweet potatoes, peeled, diced

4 tablespoons of butter

1 cup yellow onion, chopped

1 cup red bell pepper, chopped

Fresh parsley, chopped for garnish

Directions:

1.   Set your instant pot to the sauté mode, add the butter and heat it. Add the chicken and stir, cooking for 5minutes browning all sides of the chicken.

2.   Add the bell pepper, and onion, continue to cook for an additional 3minutes, stir.

3.   Add the chicken stock and sweet potatoes, set the instant pot to the Meat/Stew setting for 35minutes.

4.   Release the pressure naturally for 10minutes, once the cooking is completed.

5.   Divide into serving dishes, and garnish with parsley. Serve warm!

Instant Pot Chicken Bean Chili

Preparation Time: 35 minutes

Servings: 6

Ingredients:

1 lb. chicken, boneless, skinless, cubed

1 medium, yellow onion, diced

2 cups vegetable stock

1 15ounce can of black beans, rinsed, drained

2 cups salsa

2 tablespoons olive oil

Directions:

1.   Set your instant pot to the sauté mode, add the oil and heat it.

2.   Add the cubed chicken to instant pot, and brown on all sides for 5minutes, stir often.

3.   Add the remaining ingredients to instant pot and stir.

4.　　Close the lid place instant pot on the Bean/Chili setting for 30minutes.

5.　　Release the pressure naturally for 15minutes. Divide among serving bowls. Serve hot!

Instant Pot Herbal Chicken

Ingredients:

1 lb. chicken, cubed

2 cups chicken stock

3 tablespoons rosemary leaves, fresh, chopped

3 tablespoons thyme leaves, fresh, chopped

3 garlic cloves, minced

Salt and black pepper to taste

1 red bell pepper, chopped

1 green bell pepper, chopped

1 cup broccoli, florets

Directions:

1.　　Blend the garlic and herbs, and rub the mixture over your chicken chunks. In your instant pot heat olive oil with the sauté mode setting.

2.   Add the chicken into instant pot, stir and cook for 5minutes, browning chicken on all sides.

3.   Add the chicken stock and veggies, and close the lid on your instant pot. Set to Poultry setting for 35minutes.

4.   Release the pressure naturally for 10minutes.

5.   Divide into serving dishes. Serve warm!

Instant Pot Chicken Fillets

Preparation Time: 45 minutes

Servings: 4

Ingredients:

1 lb. chicken fillets, cut into four equal portions

¼ cup sour cream, reduced fat

2 teaspoons lemon juice

2 tablespoons stoneground mustard

Salt and pepper to taste

Lime wedges for garnish

Directions:

1.	Place the chicken fillets into your instant pot. Make a paste with the remaining ingredients except the lime wedges.

2.	Spread the mixture over the chicken fillets. Set the instant pot to the Poultry setting for 45minutes.

3.	Release the pressure naturally for 10minutes.

4.	Divide among serving plates, and garnish with lemon wedges.

Buttery Chicken with Macadamia

Ingredients:

1lb. chicken breast,

sliced into four equal portions

2 tablespoons macadamia nuts, toasted

¼ teaspoon chili powder

2 tablespoons lime juice + ½ teaspoon lime zest

2 tablespoons butter

Directions:

1.   Set your instant pot to the sauté setting, add the butter and heat it. Season the chicken with salt and black pepper.

2.   Add the chicken to instant pot and cook for 5minutes or until the chicken is slightly brown in color on all sides.

3.   Set on the Poultry setting on low for 17minutes. Release the pressure naturally for 10minutes.

4.   Make a mixture using the melted butter from instant pot, lime juice, chili powder, lime zest and pour over the chicken on serving plates.

5.   Add the toasted macadamia nuts as garnish. Serve warm!

Mushroom & Chicken Hash

Ingredients:

2 cups cooked chicken, cubed

4 tablespoons butter

4 celery ribs, finely chopped

1 medium yellow onion, diced

1 lb. button mushrooms, sliced

Directions:

1.   Set your instant pot to the sauté mode, add the butter and heat. Add the mushrooms and sauté for 2minutes.

2.   Add the onion, chicken, and celery, stir and cook for an additional 3minutes. Close the lid and set instant pot on the Poultry setting for 35minutes.

3.   Release the pressure for 10minutes.

4.   Divide into serving plates. Serve warm!

Cheesy Spinach Stuffed Chicken Breasts

Ingredients:

2 chicken breasts

1 teaspoon onion powder

1 teaspoon garlic powder

2 cups baby spinach

3 tablespoons coconut oil

1 cup parmesan cheese, shredded

1 cup mozzarella cheese, shredded

1 red bell pepper, chopped

2 cups water

Sea salt and black pepper to taste

Directions:

1.   Cover your instant pot trivet with foil. Set your instant pot to the sauté mode, add 2 tablespoons of the coconut oil and heat it.

2.   Add the chicken and brown on all sides for 5minutes. Remove the chicken, and allow to cool.

3.   Press the Keep Warm/Cancel button to end the sauté mode. In a mixing bowl, combine parmesan cheese, red pepper, mozzarella cheese, remaining 1 tablespoon of coconut oil, baby spinach and seasoning.

4.   When the chicken is cool, cut down the middle, but do not cut all the way through. Stuff with spinach mixture.

5.   Pour 2 cups of water in the instant pot. Place the trivet inside. Place the chicken on trivet. Close and seal lid.

6.   Press the Manual setting, and cook on high pressure for 7minutes. Release the pressure naturally for 10minutes.

7.   Allow the chicken to rest for 5minutes. Divide among serving plates. Serve warm!

Thyme Flavored Turkey and Squash Pie

Ingredients:

1 cup cooked and shredded Turkey Meat

½ cup chopped Kale

¼ tsp Garlic Powder

2 cups Chicken Stock

1 tsp Thyme

¼ tsp Paprika

¼ tsp Xanthan Gum

½ cup chopped Squash

½ cup shredded Cheddar Cheese

Salt and Pepper, to taste

Crust:

1 Egg

¼ cup Ghee

2 cups Almond Flour

¼ tsp Xanthan Gum

¼ cup shredded Cheddar Cheese

1/8 tsp Salt

Directions:

1.   Pour the stock into a saucepan and heat over medium heat.

2.   Add squash and turkey and cook for about 10 minutes.

3.   Stir in cheddar, kale, thyme, and the spices.

4.   Spoon out about ½ cup of the stock and whisk the xanthan gum in it.

5.   Whisk the mixture into the pot.

6.   Remove from the heat and set aside.

7.   Preheat your oven to 350 degrees.

8.   Combine all of the crust ingredients until a ball of dough is formed.

9.   Roll into a circle.

10.   Spread the turkey filling into a greased pie pan.

11.   Top with the crust.

12.   Bake for about 35 minutes.

13.   Allow to cool before serving.

14.   Enjoy!

Chicken with a TomatoAnchovy Sauce

Ingredients:

1 Red Onion, chopped

1 pound Tomatoes, chopped

4 Garlic Cloves, minced

4 Chicken Breasts, boneless and skinless

¼ cup Olive Oil

½ cup Olives, chopped

4 Anchovy Fillets, chopped

1 tbsp Capers

½ tsp Red Pepper Flakes

Salt and Pepper, to taste

Directions:

1.   Preheat your oven to 450 degrees F.

2.   Season the chicken with salt and pepper.

3.	Heat half of the oil in a pan and cook the chicken until no longer pink. About 23 minutes per side.

4.	Arrange the chicken on a lined baking sheet and place in the oven.

5.	Bake for about 8 minutes.

6.	Heat the remaining oil in the same pan.

7.	Add the rest of the ingredients.

8.	Cook for about 3 minutes.

9.	Serve the chicken topped with the sauce.

10.	Enjoy!

Chicken Casserole the Mexican Way

Ingredients:

1 tbsp Olive Oil

1 cup Red Enchilada Sauce

2 Keto Tortillas

2 Jalapenos, chopped

2 Chipotle Peppers, chopped

¼ cup Heavy Cream

1 pound boneless and skinless Chicken Thighs, chopped

4 ounces Cream Cheese

2 tbsp chopped Cilantro

½ Onion, chopped

Salt and Pepper, to taste

Directions:

1.   Heat the oil in a pan over medium heat.

2.   Add the peppers and cook for a minute.

3.   Add onion and cook until soft, or about 5 minutes.

4.   Stir in heavy cream and cream cheese, and cook until the cheese is fully melted.

5.   Meanwhile, preheat your oven to 350 degrees F.

6.   Stir the chicken, salt, pepper, and enchilada sauce, into the cheesy mixture. Set aside.

7.   Grease a baking dish with cooking spray.

8.   Arrange the tortillas at the bottom.

9.   Pour the chicken mixture over and spread it out evenly. Sprinkle with the cheeses.

10.   Cover with foil and cook for 15 minutes.

11.   Uncover, and bake for 15 minutes more.

12.   Serve sprinkled with fresh cilantro.

13.   Enjoy!

Baked Lemony Chicken

Ingredients:

1 Whole Chicken, cut into pieces

Juice and Zest of 2 Lemons

Salt and Pepper, to taste

Directions:

1.   Preheat your oven to 375 degrees F.

2.   Place all of the ingredients in a greased baking dish.

3.   Toss with your hands to combine.

4.   Place in the oven and bake for 45 minutes.

5.   Serve the chicken drizzled with the lemony cooking liquid.

6.   Enjoy!

Creamy Chicken with Paprika and Onions

Ingredients:

1 tbsp Lime Juice

2 tsp Paprika

2 tbsp Green Onions, chopped

1 ½ cups chopped yellow Onions

3 ½ pounds Chicken Breasts, boneless and skinless

1 tbsp Coconut Oil

1 cup Chicken Stock

1 tsp Red Pepper Flakes

¼ cup Coconut Milk

Salt and Pepper, to taste

Directions:

1.   Melt the coconut oil in a pan over medium heat.

2.   Add the chicken and cook for about 2 minutes per side. Transfer to a plate.

3.   Spry some cooking spray in the pan if needed, and cook the onions for 4 minutes.

4.   Stir in the remaining ingredients.

5.   After a minute or so, return the chicken to the pan.

6.   Cover the pan, reduce the heat, and cook for 15 minutes.

7.   Serve and enjoy!

Lime and Cumin Chicken Fajitas

Ingredients:

1 tsp Garlic Powder

1 tsp Sweet Paprika

2 tsp Cumin

2 tbsp Coconut Oil

2 tbsp Lime Juice

1 Red Bell pepper sliced

1 Green Bell Pepper, sliced

1 Avocado, sliced

1 tsp ground Coriander

1 tsp Chili Powder

2 pounds Chicken Breasts, cut into strips

1 tbsp chopped Cilantro

2 Limes, cut into wedges

Salt and Pepper, to taste

Directions:

1. Combine the lime juice with the spices, in a bowl.

2. Add the chicken strips and coat well.

3. Melt half of the coconut oil in a pan over medium heat.

4. Add the chicken and cook for about 3 minutes per side. Transfer to a plate.

5. Melt the remaining coconut oil.

6. Add onion and peppers and cook for 56 minutes.

7. Return the chicken and season with salt and pepper, if desired.

8. Serve the chicken topped with avocado slices and lime wedges, and sprinkled with cilantro.

9. Enjoy!

Tarragon Chicken with Mushrooms

Ingredients:

1 tsp Dijon Mustard

4 Chicken Thighs

2 cups sliced Mushrooms

1 tbsp chopped tarragon

¼ cup Ghee

½ tsp Onion Powder

½ tsp Garlic Powder

Salt and Pepper, to taste

½ cup Water

Directions:

1.   Melt half of the ghee in a pan over medium heat.

2.   Season the chicken thighs with some salt and pepper, and cook them for 3 minutes per side. Transfer to a plate.

3.   Melt the remaining ghee in the same pan and cook the mushrooms for 5 minutes.

4.   Stir in water and mustard.

5.   Return the chicken to the pan, reduce the heat, and cook covered for 15 minutes.

6.   Uncover, stir in the tarragon, and cook for 5 more minutes.

7.   Serve and enjoy!

Chicken Breasts in an Olive Sauce

Ingredients:

2 tbsp Coconut Oil

1 Chicken Breast, cut into 4 pieces

3 Garlic Cloves, crushed

1 cup pitted Black Olives

2 tbsp Olive Oil

1 tbsp Lemon Juice

¼ cup Parsley

¼ tsp Salt

Pinch of Black Pepper

Directions:

1.   Place the olives, salt, pepper, olive oil, parsley, and lemon juice, in your food processor.

2.	Pulse until smooth.

3.	Melt the coconut oil in a skillet.

4.	Add garlic and cook for 12 minutes. Discard.

5.	Add the chicken to the skillet and cook for about 34 minutes on each side.

6.	Serve the chicken topped with the olive sauce.

7.	njoy!

Sweet and OrangeFlavored Duck Breast with Spinach

Ingredients:

1 tbsp Swerve

1 medium Duck Breast

1 cup Baby Spinach

2 tbsp Ghee

1 tbsp Heavy Cream

¼ tsp Sage

½ tsp Orange Extract

Directions:

1.	Melt the ghee in a pan over medium heat.

2.   Add swerve and cook until it caramelizes.

3.   Stir in the orange extract and cook for a minute or so.

4.   Whisk in the heavy cream. Let simmer gently.

5.   Heat another pan over medium heat and coat it with cooking spray.

6.   Add the duck and cook for 4 minutes per side.

7.   Add the spinach to the orange mixture and cook until it wilts.

8.   Stir in the sage and set aside.

9.   When the duck is cooked, transfer it to a plate.

10.   Pour the sauce over it.

11.   Serve and enjoy!

Garlicky Chicken Nuggets

Ingredients:

1 Egg, beaten

½ cup Ghee

2 Chicken Breasts, cut into cubes

2 tbsp Garlic Powder

½ cup Coconut Flour

Salt and Pepper, to taste

Directions:

1.   Place the coconut flour, garlic powder, and some salt and pepper in a bowl. Stir to combine.

2.   Dip the chicken pieces in egg first, and then coat with the coconut/garlic mixture.

3.   Melt the ghee in a pan over medium heat.

4.   Cook the chicken nuggets for about 5 minutes on each side.

5.   Drain on paper towels before serving.

6.   Enjoy!

Chapter 15: Keto Seafood

Calamari with Sriracha Sauce

Ingredients:

1 squid, cut into medium rings

¼ tsp cayenne pepper

1 egg, whisked

2 tbsp coconut flour

Salt and black pepper to taste

Coconut oil, for frying

1 tbsp lemon juice

4 tbsp mayo

1 tsp sriracha sauce

Directions:

1.   Season squid rings with salt, pepper, and cayenne, and put themin a bowl.

2.   In a separate bowl, whisk the egg with salt, pepper and coconut flour.

3.   Dredge calamari rings in the egg mix.

4.　　　Heat a pan with enough coconut oil to cover the surface over medium heat. Fry the calamari rings until they become gold on both sides.

5.　　　Transfer to paper towels, drain grease, and put in a bowl.

6.　　　In another bowl, mix mayonnaise with lemon juice and sriracha sauce, and serve your calamari rings with this sauce on the side.

7.　　　Enjoy!

Shrimp and Calamari Dippers

Ingredients:

8 oz calamari, cut into medium rings

7 oz shrimp, peeled and deveined

1 egg

3 tbsp coconut flour

1 tbsp coconut oil

2 tbsp avocado, chopped

1 tsp tomato paste

1 tbsp mayonnaise

¼ tsp Worcestershire sauce

1 tsp lemon juice

2 lemon slices

Salt and black pepper to taste

½ tsp turmeric

Directions:

1.   In a bowl, whisk the egg with coconut oil.

2.   Toss the calamari and shrimp in the bowl to coat them.

3.   In a new bowl, mix the flour with salt, pepper, and turmeric.

4.   Dredge the calamari and shrimp in this flour mix, place everything on a lined baking sheet, and bake in the oven at 400 degrees F for 10 minutes.

5.   Flip calamari and shrimp to their other side, and bake for 10 minutes more.

6.   Meanwhile, in a bowl, mash avocado with mayo and tomato paste using a fork.

7.   Add Worcestershire sauce, lemon juice, salt and pepper to the avocado bowl.

8.   Divide baked calamari and shrimp onto plates, and serve with the sauce and lemon slices on the side.

9.   Enjoy!

Fresh Salad with Octopus

Ingredients:

21 oz octopus, rinsed

Juice of 1 lemon

4 celery stalks, chopped

3 oz olive oil

Salt and black pepper to taste

4 tbsp parsley, chopped

Directions:

1.   Place the octopus in a pot, add water until it's covered, and bring to a boil over medium heat. Cook for 40 minutes, covered, drain, and leave aside to cool down when done.

2.   Chop cooled octopus, and put it in a salad bowl.

3.   Add celery stalks, parsley, olive oil and lemon juice, and toss everything together well.

4.   Season with salt and pepper, toss once more, and serve.

5.   Enjoy!

Classic Clam Chowder Soup

Ingredients:

1 cup celery stalks, chopped

Salt and black pepper to taste

1 tsp dried thyme

2 cups chicken stock

14 oz canned baby clams

2 cups heavy cream

1 cup onion, chopped

13 bacon slices, chopped

Directions:

1.   Brown bacon in a pan over medium high heat, and transfer the cooked pieces to a bowl. Save the grease in the pan.

2.   Heat up the same pan over medium heat, add celery and onion, and cook for 5 minutes.

3.   Transfer cooked and remaining ingredients to a slow cooker, and cook on high heat for 2 hours.

4.   Divide into bowls and serve.

5.   Enjoy!

Fish Stew Recipe

Ingredients:

2 lbspollock fillets; skinless

1 lb king prawns; raw shelled

3 garlic cloves; crushed

3 cups fish stock

1/2 cup extra virgin olive oil

2 small onions; finely chopped.

2 celery stalks; finely chopped.

1 cup fresh parsley; finely chopped.

1 tbsp fresh rosemary; finely chopped.

1 tsp sea salt

Directions:

1.   Plug in the instant pot and grease the inner pot with three tablespoons of olive oil

2.   Add onions and crushed garlic. Press the *Sauté* button and cook for 4 - 5 minutes, stirring constantly

3.   Now; add the remaining ingredients and stir all well. Press the *Cancel'* button to turn off the *Sauté* mode

4.   Seal the lid and set the steam release handle. Press the *Manual* button and set the timer for 10 minutes.

5.   When done; press the *Cancel'* button again and perform a quick pressure release by moving the pressure valve to the *Venting* position.

6.   Carefully open the lid and sprinkle the stew with some freshly squeezed lemon juice before serving.

Chili Hake Fillets

Ingredients:

2 lbs hake fillets; skinless

3 garlic cloves; minced

1/4 cup soy sauce

3 cups fish stock

1/2 cup olive oil

1/4 cup apple cider vinegar

1 red onion; finely chopped.

2 tbsp fresh dill; finely chopped.

2 tsp chili powder

2 tsp fresh rosemary

1 tsp sea salt

Directions:

1.   Rinse fillets under cold running water and place them in a deep bowl. Drizzle with olive oil and apple cider vinegar. Sprinkle with rosemary, salt, dill, and chili powder. Cover with the lid and set aside

2.   Plug in the instant pot and grease the inner pot with some oil. Press the *Sauté* button and add onions and garlic. Stir-fry for 3 - 4 minutes and season with some salt and optionally some pepper

3.   Remove the fillets from the bowl and place in the pot. Drizzle with about two tablespoons of the marinade and pour in the stock. Seal the lid and set the steam release handle

4.	Press the *Manual* button and set the timer for 12 minutes on *High* pressure

5.	When done; perform a quick release and carefully open the lid. Press the *Sauté* button and pour in the soy sauce

6.	Gently stir again and cook for 3 - 4 minutes. Turn off the pot and serve immediately

Flounder with Seafood Étouffée

Ingredients:

For the seasoning:

2 tsp onion powder

2 tsp thyme, dried

2 tsp sweet paprika

2 tsp garlic powder

Salt and black pepper to taste

½ tsp allspice, ground

1 tsp oregano, dried

A pinch of cayenne pepper

¼ tsp nutmeg, ground

¼ tsp cloves

A pinch of cinnamon powder

For the etouffee:

2 shallots, chopped

1 tbsp ghee

8 oz bacon, sliced

1 green bell pepper, chopped

1 celery stick, chopped

2 tbsp coconut flour

1 tomato, chopped

4 garlic cloves, minced

8 oz shrimp, peeled, deveined and chopped

2 cups chicken stock

1 tbsp coconut milk

A handful parsley, chopped

1 tsp Tabasco sauce

Salt and black pepper to taste

For the flounder:

4 flounder fillets

2 tbsp ghee

Directions:

1.   For the seasoning, combine all spices in a bowl and mix together.

2.   Reserve 2 tablespoons of this mix, and rub the flounder with the rest.

3.   Heat up a pot over medium heat, and cook the bacon for 6 minutes.

4.   Add celery, bell pepper, shallots and 1 tablespoon ghee to the pot, and cook for 4 minutes.

5.   Add tomato and garlic, and cook for 4 minutes.

6.   Add coconut flour and reserved seasoning, stir, and cook for an additional 2 minutes.

7.   Pour in chicken stock and bring the pot to a simmer.

8.   Meanwhile, heat up a pan with 2 tablespoons ghee over medium high heat, add the flounder, and cook for 2 minutes on each side. Set this pan aside.

9.   Add shrimp to the pot of stock, stir, and cook for 2 minutes.

10.   Add parsley, salt, pepper, coconut milk and Tabasco sauce to the pot, then take off heat.

11.   Divide fish onto plates, top with the shrimp sauce, and serve.

12.   Enjoy!

Chopped Shrimp Tarragon Salad

Ingredients:

2 tbsp olive oil

1 lb shrimp, peeled and deveined

Salt and black pepper to taste

2 tbsp lime juice

3 endives, leaves separated

3 tbsp parsley, chopped

2 tsp mint, chopped

1 tbsp tarragon, chopped

1 tbsp lemon juice

2 tbsp mayonnaise

1 tsp lime zest

½ cup sour cream

Directions:

1.   In a bowl, mix the shrimp with salt, pepper, and olive oil. Toss to coat, and then spread the shrimp on a lined baking sheet.

2.   Place the shrimp in the oven at 400 degrees F, and bake for 10 minutes.

3.   After baking, squeeze on lime juice, toss to coat the shrimp again, and leave aside for now.

4.   In a new bowl, mix mayo with sour cream, lime zest, lemon juice, salt, pepper, tarragon, mint and parsley.

5.   Chop the shrimp, add to salad dressing, and toss to coat everything. Spoon the salad into endive leaves.

6.   Serve right away.

7.   Enjoy!

Spicy Saucy Oysters

Ingredients:

12 oysters, shucked

Juice of 1 lemon

Juice from 1 orange

Zest from 1 orange

Juice from 1 lime

Zest from 1 lime

2 tbsp ketchup

1 Serrano chili pepper, chopped

1 cup tomato juice

½ tsp ginger, grated

¼ tsp garlic, minced

Salt to taste

¼ cup olive oil

¼ cup cilantro, chopped

¼ cup scallions, chopped

Directions:

1.   In a bowl, combine all ingredients, except for oysters, with a whisk.

2.   Spoon this mixture into oysters, and serve them immediately.

3.   Enjoy!

Creamy Lobster Soup

Ingredients:

4 garlic cloves, minced

1 small red onion, chopped

24 oz lobster chunks, precooked

Salt and black pepper to taste

½ cup tomato paste

2 carrots, finely chopped

4 celery stalks, chopped

1 quart seafood stock

1 tbsp olive oil

1 cup heavy cream

3 bay leaves

1 tsp thyme, dried

1 tsp peppercorns

1 tsp paprika

1 tsp xanthan gum

¼ cup parsley, chopped

1 tbsp lemon juice

Directions:

1.   Heat up a large pot with the olive oil over medium heat, add onion, and cook for 4 minutes.

2.   Add garlic, stir, and cook for 1 minute.

3.   Add celery and carrot, stir, and cook for another minute.

4.   Add tomato paste and stock to the pot.

5.   Add bay leaves, salt, pepper, peppercorns, paprika, thyme and xanthan gum. Stir the ingredients, and simmer over medium heat for 1 hour.

6.   Discard bay leaves, pour in cream, and bring to a simmer.

7.   Use an immersion blender to combine the ingredients, and add lobster chunks.

8.   Cook for a few minutes more.

9.   Stir in lemon juice, divide into bowls, and sprinkle parsley on top.

10.   Enjoy!

Salmon Nori Rolls

Ingredients:

2 nori sheets

1 small avocado, pitted and finely chopped

6 oz smoked salmon. Sliced

4 oz cream cheese

1 cucumber, sliced

1 tsp wasabi paste

Pickled ginger for serving

Directions:

1.   Place nori sheets flat on a sushi mat.

2.   Divide salmon slices among the sheets. Then divide the avocado and cucumber slices.

3.   In a bowl, mix the cream cheese with wasabi paste and stir well to combine.

4.   Spread the mix over cucumber slices, and roll your nori sheets. Slice each sheet into 6 pieces, and serve with pickled ginger.

5.   Enjoy!

Citrus Pepper and Salmon Skewers

Ingredients:

12 oz salmon fillet, cubed

1 red onion, cut into chunks

½ red bell pepper, cut in chunks

½ green bell pepper, cut in chunks

½ orange bell pepper, cut in chunks

Juice from 1 lemon

Salt and black pepper to taste

1 tbsp olive oil

Directions:

1.   Thread skewers with onion, the bell pepper, and salmon cubes evenly.

2.   Season the skewers with salt and pepper. Drizzle olive oil and lemon juice over them, and place them on preheated grill on medium high heat.

3.   Cook for 4 minutes on each side, divide between plates, and serve.

4.   Enjoy!

Swordfish Steaks with Salsa

Ingredients:

2 medium swordfish steaks

Salt and black pepper to taste

2 tsp avocado oil

1 tbsp cilantro, chopped

1 mango, chopped

1 avocado, pitted, and chopped

¼ tsp cumin

¼ tsp onion powder

¼ tsp garlic powder

1 orange, peeled and sliced

½ tbsp balsamic vinegar

Directions:

1.   Season the swordfish steaks with salt, pepper, garlic powder, onion powder and cumin on each side.

2.   Heat a pan with half of the olive oil over medium high heat, add fish steaks, and cook them for 3 minutes on each side.

3. Meanwhile, in a clean bowl, mix the avocado with mango, cilantro, balsamic vinegar, salt, pepper and the rest of the olive oil.

4. Divide fish on two plates, top with mango salsa, and serve with orange slices on the side.

5. Enjoy!

Tuna and Cauliflower Salad

Ingredients:

For the Tuna

1 ahi tuna steak

2 tbsp coconut oil

1 cauliflower head, florets separated

2 tbsp green onions, chopped

1 avocado, pitted and chopped

1 cucumber, grated

1 nori sheet, torn

For the salad dressing:

1 tbsp sesame oil

2 tbsp coconut aminos

1 tbsp apple cider vinegar

A pinch of salt

1 tsp stevia

Directions:

1.   Put cauliflower florets in your food processor, and pulse until you obtain a cauliflower "rice".

2.   Fill a pot with water, add a steamer basket inside, and put the cauliflower rice inside. Bring the water to a boil over medium heat, cover, steam for a few minutes, drain, and transfer "rice" to a bowl.

3.   Heat a pan with the coconut oil over medium high heat, and add the tuna steak. Cook for 1 minute on each side, and transfer to a cutting board.

4.   Divide cauliflower rice into bowls, top with nori pieces, cucumber, green onions and avocado.

5.   For the dressing, in a bowl, mix all ingredients with a whisk.

6.   Drizzle this over cauliflower rice and mixed veggies, top with tuna pieces and serve.

7.   Enjoy!

Savory Seasoned Swordfish

Ingredients:

1 tbsp parsley, chopped

1 lemon, cut into wedges

4 swordfish steaks

3 garlic cloves, minced

1/3 cup chicken stock

3 tbsp olive oil

¼ cup lemon juice

Salt and black pepper to taste

½ tsp rosemary, dried

½ tsp sage, dried

½ tsp marjoram, dried

Directions:

1.   In a bowl, whisk together the chicken stock with garlic, lemon juice, olive oil, salt, pepper, sage, marjoram and rosemary.

2.   Add swordfish steaks to the bowl, toss to coat, and keep in the fridge to marinate for 3 hours.

3.   Place marinated fish steaks on preheated grill over medium high heat, and cook for 5 minutes on each side.

4.   Serve on plates with parsley and lemon wedges on the side.

5.   Enjoy!

Classic Crab Cakes

Ingredients:

1 lb crabmeat

¼ cup parsley, chopped

Salt and black pepper to taste

2 green onions, chopped

¼ cup cilantro, chopped

1 tsp jalapeno pepper, minced

1 tsp lemon juice

1 tsp Worcestershire sauce

1 tsp old bay seasoning

½ tsp mustard powder

½ cup mayonnaise

1 egg

2 tbsp olive oil

Directions:

1. In a large bowl, mix the crab meat with salt, pepper, parsley, green onions, cilantro, jalapeno, lemon juice, old bay seasoning, mustard powder and Worcestershire sauce with a large spoon or spatula.

2. In another bowl, mix egg wit mayo with a whisk.

3. Combine this mix with the crabmeat mix, and stir everything.

4. Shape 6 patties from this mix with your hands, and place them on a plate.

5. Heat a large pan with the olive oil over medium high heat, and add 3 crab cakes. Cook for 3 minutes per side, and transfer them to paper towels.

6. Repeat with the other 3 crab cakes, drain excess grease, and serve immediately.

7. Enjoy!

Tilapia Bites

Ingredients:

1 pound Tilapia Fillets

3 Eggs

3 tbsp. Olive Oil

½ cup Half and Half

1 tsp Red Pepper Flakes

1 tsp Coriander

Juice of 1 Lemon

1 tsp Lemon Zest

¼ tsp Pepper

2 tbsp. ground Almonds

Directions:

1.   Whisk together the eggs, spices, zest, and almond flour.

2.   Heat the oil in the IP on SAUTE.

3.   Chop the tilapia and dip into the egg mixture.

4.   Cook on SAUTE until golden.

5.   Pour the lemon juice and half and half over and close the lid.

6.   Cook on HIGH for 2 minutes.

7.   Do a quick pressure release.

8.   Serve and enjoy!

Lemon Pepper Wild Alaskan Cod

Ingredients:

8 ounces Wild Alaskan Cod

¼ tsp Garlic Powder

1 tsp Lemon Pepper

4 Lemon Sliced

1 tbsp. Olive Oil

2 tbsp. Butter, melted

1 ½ cups Water

Directions:

1.   Pour the water into the Instant Pot.

2.   Cut the cod in half and place each half on top of an aluminum foil piece.

3.   Season with garlic powder and lemon pepper.

4.   Top with the lemon slices, drizzle with oil, and wrap in foil.

5.   Place into the steamer basket.

6.   Close the lid and cook on HIGH for 6 minutes.

7.   Unwrap and drizzle with melted butter.

8.   Serve and enjoy!

White Fish in Ginger Orange Sauce

Ingredients:

4 White Fish Fillets

1 1inch piece of Ginger, sliced

Juice and Zest of 1 Orange

1 cup White Wine

3 Spring Onions, chopped

1 tbsp. Olive Oil

Salt and Pepper, to taste

Directions:

1.   Combine the juice, zest, wine, ginger, and spring onions in the Instant Pot.

2.   Drizzle the fish with olive oil and sprinkle with some salt and pepper.

3.   Rub to coat well.

4.   Place in the steamer basket.

5.   Lower the basket into the pot and close the lid.

6. Cook on HIGH for 6 minutes.

7. Do a quick pressure release.

8. Serve and enjoy!

Tomato Tuna Pasta

Ingredients:

1 Tuna Can, drained

1 cup canned diced Tomatoes

1 tsp minced Garlic

1 tbsp. diced Onions

1 tbsp. chopped Parsley

3 tbsp. grated Parmesan Cheese

2 cups Zucchini Noodles

¼ cup Tomato Sauce

1 tbsp. Butter

Directions:

1. Melt the butter in the Instant Pot on SAUTE.

2. Add onions and garlic and cook for 2 minutes.

3.   Add tomatoes and tomato sauce and cook for 2 more minutes.

4.   Stir in the remaining ingredients, except the cheese.

5.   Close the lid and cook on HIGH for 3 minutes.

6.   Do a quick pressure release.

7.   Sprinkle with parmesan cheese.

8.   Serve and enjoy!

Salmon on a Veggie Bed

Ingredients:

4 Salmon Fillets

3 tsp Olive Oil

½ Lemon, sliced

1 Bell Pepper, julienned

1 Zucchini, julienned

1 Carrot, julienned

1 Tarragon Sprig

A handful of parsley

A handful of Basil

1 cup of Water

Directions:

1.   Pour the water into the Instant Pot and place the herbs inside.

2.   Arrange the veggies on the rack.

3.   Top with the salmon filletsskin side down.

4.   Drizzle with oil and top with lemon sliced.

5.   Close the lid and cook on HIGH for 5 minutes.

6.   Do a quick pressure release.

7.   Serve and enjoy!

Conclusion

I do hope that this book has been helpful and you found the information contained within the chapters useful!

For those who have already been able to make the mental conversion to change, then I trust, that you will find this a far more accessible and easy to maintain eating method than those you may have tackled in the past. I am convinced that just a few weeks on the Ketogenic diet will produce such good results that you will be encouraged to turn it into a permanent way of life.

Keep in mind that you are not only limited to the recipes provided in this book! Just go ahead and keep on exploring until you create your very own culinary masterpiece!

Stay healthy and stay safe!

www.ingramcontent.com/pod-product-compliance
Lightning Source LLC
Chambersburg PA
CBHW060311030426
42336CB00011B/997